Clinics in Human Lactation

Hospital Breastfeeding Issues:

Hypoglycemia, Jaundice, and Supplementation

Nancy E. Wight, MD, IBCLC, FABM, FAAP

© 2012
Neonatologist, San Diego Neonatology, Inc.
Medical Director, Sharp HealthCare Lactation Service
Sharp Mary Birch Hospital for Women & Newborns
3003 Health Center Drive
San Diego, California 92123

Hospital Breastfeeding Issues:

Hypoglycemia, Jaundice And Supplementation

Praeclarus Press, LLC
2504 Sweetgum Lane
Amarillo, Texas 79124 USA
806-367-9950
www.PraeclarusPress.com

DISCLAIMER
The information contained in this publication is advisory only and is not intended to replace sound clinical judgment or individualized patient care. The author disclaims all warranties, whether expressed or implied, including any warranty as the quality, accuracy, safety, or suitability of this information for any particular purpose.

ISBN: 978-1-939807-62-5

Table of Contents

Learning Objectives

At the conclusion of the monograph, the reader will be able to:

1. Describe the normal newborn breastfeeding course in regards to feeding behavior, weight loss and gain, and stool progression.

2. Describe a breastfeeding-supportive approach for treatment of hypoglycemia.

3. Outline the breastfeeding-supportive management of jaundice in the breastfed infant.

4. Discuss appropriate supplementation for the hypoglycemic or jaundiced infant.

5. Recognize how some current hospital policies and practices may interfere with optimal breastfeeding.

Introduction

"A pair of mammary glands has the advantage over the two hemispheres of the most learned professor's mind in the art of compounding nutritious fluid for infants."

Oliver Wendell Holmes (Sr.) 1809–1894

In the United States, most pregnant women plan to breastfeed (DiGirolamo, Thompson, Martorell, Fein, & Grummer-Strawn, 2005), and nearly all births occur in the hospital setting (Hamilton, Martin, & Ventura, 2009). However, there is a major gap between women's intentions to breastfeed and the number of women who actually leave the hospital breastfeeding. There is an even larger gap between *any* breastfeeding and *exclusive* breastfeeding at hospital discharge (Figure I.1).

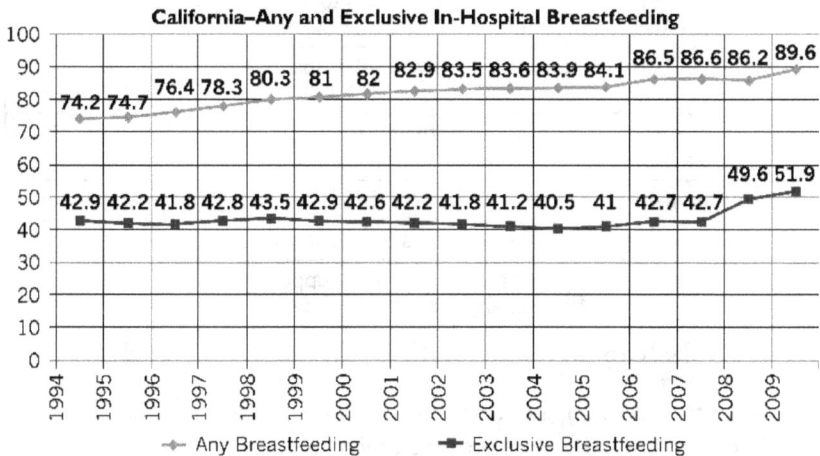

California–Any and Exclusive In-Hospital Breastfeeding

Any Breastfeeding values (1994–2009): 74.2, 74.7, 76.4, 78.3, 80.3, 81, 82, 82.9, 83.5, 83.6, 83.9, 84.1, 86.5, 86.6, 86.2, 89.6

Exclusive Breastfeeding values: 42.9, 42.2, 41.8, 42.8, 43.5, 42.9, 42.6, 42.2, 41.8, 41.2, 40.5, 41, 42.7, 42.7, 49.6, 51.9

Figure I.1. California–Any and Exclusive In-Hospital Breastfeeding: 1994–2010 Excludes records with feeding 'not reported.' **Data Source:** California Department of Health Services, Genetic Disease Branch, Newborn Screening Database.

Hospital practices and policies in maternity settings can create barriers to supporting a mother's decision to breastfeed, and to breastfeed exclusively (U.S. Department of Health and Human Services, 2011). National data from the Centers for Disease Control and Prevention (CDC) survey of Maternity Practices in Infant Nutrition and Care (mPINC), which assesses breastfeeding-related maternity practices in U.S. hospitals and birth centers, indicate that barriers to breastfeeding are common during labor, delivery, and postpartum care (Perrine et al., 2011). Hospital policies and practices to support breastfeeding are critical for improving breastfeeding rates. However, in 2009, only 3.5% of U.S. hospitals were following at least nine of the ten practices consistent with the Baby-Friendly Ten Steps to Successful Breastfeeding (Figure I.2; Baby-Friendly USA, 2011; Perrine et al., 2011; World Health Organization, 1989).

The Ten Steps to Successful Breastfeeding	
The BFHI promotes, protects, and supports breastfeeding through The Ten Steps to Successful Breastfeeding for Hospitals, as outlined by UNICEF/WHO.	
The steps for the United States are:	
1	Have a written breastfeeding policy that is routinely communicated to all health care staff.
2	Train all health care staff in skills necessary to implement this policy.
3	Inform all pregnant women about the benefits and management of breastfeeding.
4	Help mothers initiate breastfeeding within one hour of birth.
5	Show mothers how to breastfeed and how to maintain lactation, even if they are separated from their infants.
6	Give newborn infants no food or drink other than breastmilk, unless medically indicated.
7	Practice "rooming in"·· allow mothers and infants to remain together 24 hours a day.
8	Encourage breastfeeding on demand.
9	Give no pacifiers or artificial nipples to breastfeeding infants.
10	Foster the establishment of breastfeeding support groups and refer mothers to them on discharge from the hospital or clinic.

Figure I.2. The Ten Steps to Successful Breastfeeding (Baby-Friendly USA)

Despite an explosion of research detailing evidence-based lactation physiology and breastfeeding practices, there has been, and continues to be, considerable misinformation about the normal course of breastfeeding and how to support it. The information in medical texts is often incomplete, inconsistent, and inaccurate (Ogburn, Philipp, Espey, Merewood, & Espindola, 2011; Philipp, Merewood, Gerendas, & Baucherner, 2004). Clinicians report feeling they have insufficient knowledge and low levels of clinical competence regarding breastfeeding (Freed et al., 1995; Renfrew et al., 2006). A survey of pediatricians showed that many believe the benefits of breastfeeding do not outweigh the challenges that may be associated with it (Feldman-Winter, Schanler, O'Connor, & Lawrence, 2008). In addition, many physicians and other healthcare providers underestimate their influence on breastfeeding success (Szucs, Miracle, & Rosenman,

2009; Taveras et al., 2004). Taveras and colleagues (2004) found that clinicians' perceptions of the counseling they provided (always or usually) on breastfeeding did not match their patients' perceptions of the counseling received (infrequently or rarely). There is a very big difference between telling a mother about the benefits of breastfeeding and actively promoting and supporting breastfeeding, especially when the mother is experiencing difficulties.

Breastfeeding may be instinctive for the infant, but our current culture requires learning on the part of the mother. In the recent past role models have been few. Idyllic expectations (fed by artificial milk company marketing) have clashed with the reality of caring for a newborn, whether breastfed or not, leading to disillusionment and breastfeeding "failures." Breastfeeding "failure" includes everything from a shorter duration of breastfeeding than the mother had planned to readmissions for jaundice, dehydration, failure to thrive, and occasionally tragic deaths. The mother should define what breastfeeding "success" is for her. Our role as healthcare providers is to provide evidence-based information and management strategies to help her meet her goals.

Although breastfeeding is natural, there can be many challenges, especially when hospital policies and practices are not supportive. Most mothers are capable of breastfeeding successfully, but lactation, like all physiologic functions, sometimes fails because of various medical causes, as well as problem mismanagement. Hypoglycemia, jaundice, and supplementation are common hospital issues that may compromise breastfeeding. Managing these issues in an evidence-based and breastfeeding-supportive manner may preserve the breastfeeding relationship, extend breastfeeding duration, and improve the health of the infant, mother, and community.

Chapter 1. What is Normal?

The Physiology of Transition

Most infants are well hydrated via the placenta at birth. Urine output usually exceeds fluid intake for the first three to four days after birth. Small colostrum feedings, usually 2 to 15 ml per feeding, are:

- Physiologic and appropriate for the size of the newborn infant's stomach (Naveed, Manjunath, & Sreenivas, 1992; Scammon & Doyle, 1920; Zangen et al., 2001).

- Sufficient to prevent hypoglycemia in healthy term infants (Wight, 2006; Williams, 1997).

- Easy to manage as the infant learns to coordinate suck, swallow, and breathing.

- Enough to satisfy hunger and thirst.

- Sufficient to meet the sucking needs of the newborn, which are much greater than the quantity of food needed.

The average physiologic capacity of a newborn stomach on day one is 7 ml, and anatomic capacity (stretched volume) is 32 ml (Figure 1.1).

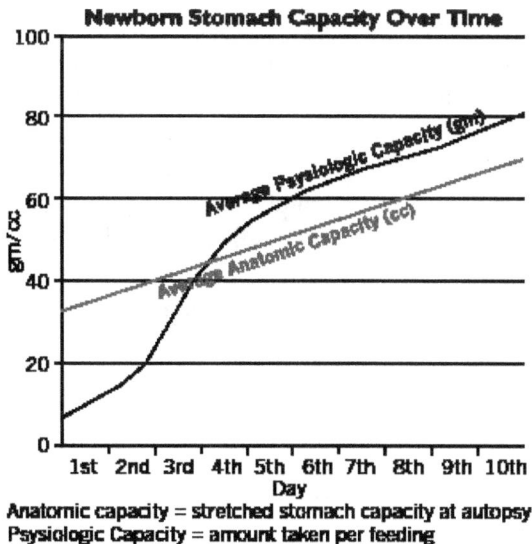

Figure 1.1. Newborn Stomach Capacity Over Time. **Source:** Scammon & Doyle, 1920. Used with permission from AMA.

Stomach capacity also varies by the size of the infant (Table 1.1; Naveed et al., 1992).

Birth weight (g)	Stretched Stomach Capacity (mL) Naveed et al, 1992					
	Stillborn		Live born		Total	
	No	Mean ± SD (Range)	No	Mean ± SD (Range)	No	Mean ± SD (Range)
500-1000	15	8.6 ± 2.4 (5-15)	6	9.5 ± 2.3 (5-12)	21	8.9 ± 2.4 (5-15)
1001-1500	12	10.6 ± 4.4 (5-20)	6	10.2 ± 2.6 (8-15)	18	10.5 ± 3.9 5-20)
1501-2000	14	11.3 ± 3.9 (5-20)	8	22.8 ± 10.0 (10-40)	22	15.5 ± 8.7 (5-40)
2001-2500	11	15.6 ± 5.4 (10-25)	8	18.1 ± 9.2 (10-30)	19	16.7 ± 7.1 (10-30)
> 2500	11	19.6 ± 7.8 (10-35)	9	17.8 ± 7.5 (10-25)	20	18.8 ± 7.6 (10-35)

Table 1.1. Stretched Stomach Capacity. Source: Reproduced with permission from the Indian Society of Gastroenterology.

During the first three postnatal days, the newborn stomach becomes more compliant and develops more receptive relaxation, associated with a larger volume capacity (Zangen et al., 2001). The small volume of colostrum and small newborn stomach correlate nicely! Why do we expect newborns to handle 30–60 ml from day one?

Milk Intake

Colostrum intake in the first few days of life has been documented in a few studies (Dollberg, Lahav, & Mimouni, 2001; Evans, Evans, Royal, Esterman, & James, 2003; Santoro, Martinez, Ricco, & Jorge, 2010). Dollberg et al. (2001) compared the intakes of breastfed (by test-weighing) and bottle-fed infants during the first two days of life. As you can see in Table 1.2, the breastfed infants had lesser intake and greater weight loss than the bottle-fed infants. However, the hospital circumstances were far from ideal, with all mothers receiving epidural anesthesia, no rooming-in, scheduled four-hour feedings, and the first feeding between two and ten hours after birth.

Characteristics of Milk Intake in Breastfed and Bottle-fed Infants			
	Breast-fed n = 15	Formula-fed n = 28	Significance
Gender (M:F)	7:8	13:15	ns
Birthweight (g)	3258 ± 408	3348 ± 348	ns
Gestational age (wks)	39.6 ± 0.9	39.7 ± 1.2	ns
Parity	2.3 ± 1.3	2.4 ± 0.9	ns
Apgar Score 1 min.	9.3 ± 0.5	9.4 ± 0.7	ns
Apgar Score 5 min.	10.0 ± 0.0	9.9 ± 0.4	ns
Weight loss day 1 (g)	149 ± 96	130 ± 56	ns
Weight loss day 2 (g)	67 ± 58	21 ± 46	$p = 0.015$
Age at first feed (h)	7.8 ± 2.6	4.9 ± 2.7	$p = 0.019$
Intake day 1 (mL/kg)	9.6 ± 10.3	18.5 ± 9.6	$p = 0.011$
Intake day 2 (mL/kg)	13.0 ± 11.3	42.2 ± 14.2	$p < 0.001$

Table 1.2. Characteristics of Milk Intake in Breastfed and Bottle-Fed Infants
Source: Dollberg S et al. J Am Coll Nutr 2001; 20(3):209–211. Reproduced with permission from the American College of Nutrition.

Evans et al. (2003) investigated the effect of cesarean section on breastmilk intakes over the first six days of life. The average intake for infants born by normal vaginal delivery (NVD) was 6 mL/kg/day and 25 mL/kg/day on days one and two, respectively. The intake for infants born by cesarean section (CS) was significantly less for days one through four. Although they did not report the number of breastfeeds per day, they concluded that the volumes of milk recommended in texts were excessive (Table 1.3).

Breastmilk transfer (mL/kg body weight) for days 1-6							
Group	Day 1	Day 2	Day 3	Day 4	Day 5	Day 6	Total days 1-6
NVD							
Mean (SE)	6 (1.4)	25 (2.2)	66 (3.6)	106 (3.9)	123 (4.5)	138 (3.9)	450 (30.4)
Number	26	88	88	88	88	88	26
CS							
Mean (SE)	4 (0.6)	13 (1.1)	44 (2)	82 (3.5)	111 (3.5)	129 (3.2)	358 (22.1)
Number	23	97	97	97	97	97	23
Unadjusted significance	0.151	<0.001	<0.001	<0.001	0.033	0.079	0.020
Adjusted significance	0.031	<0.001	0.001	<0.001	0.046	0.118	0.001

Table 1.3. Breastmilk Transfer (mL/kg) for Days 1–6 of Life. **Source**: Evans KC et al. Arch Dis Child Fetal Neonatal Ed 2003; 88:F380–382. Used with permission BMJ Publishing Group Ltd.

Finally, Santoro et al. (2010) confirmed the normal low intake in optimally breastfed infants by recording the number of breastfeeds and weight gain with each feed in the first 24 hours of life for 30 mother-infant dyads. They concluded that during the first 24 hours of life, the average breastmilk intake was 15 ± 11 g (Table 1.4).

Number of Breastfeeding and Colostrum Ingestion during the First 24 Hours of Life					
Hours of Life	Dyads	Breastfeeding (Min - Max)	P*	Weight Gain (g) (Min - Max)	P*
0-8	30	3.4 ± 0.8 (2-5)	.65	5.3 ± 3.5 (0.3-16.2)	.065
0-8	30	3.3 ± 1.0 (2-5)	.65	3.7 ± 2.6 (0.6-11.9)	.065
0-8	30	3.5 ± 1.1 (0-6)	.65	6.0 ± 4.9 (0.0-17.6)	.065
* One-way analysis of variance.					

Table 1.4. Colostrum Intake During the First Day of Life. Source: Santoro et al. J Peds 2010; 156(1): 29-32. Used with permission from Elsevier.

Newborn Weight Loss and Gain

Healthy term infants have sufficient body water to meet their metabolic needs, even in hot climates (Cohen, Brown, Rivera, & Dewey, 2000; Goldberg & Adams, 1983; Marchini & Stock, 1997; Rodriquez et al., 2000; Sachdev, Krishna, & Puri, 1992; Sachdev, Krishna, Puri, Satyanarayana, & Kumar, 1991; Shrago, 1987). Fluid necessary to replace insensible fluid loss is adequately provided by breastmilk alone (American Academy of Pediatrics Section on Breastfeeding, 2012; Sachdev et al., 1991; Scariati, Grummer-Strawn, & Fein, 1997). Newborns lose weight due to physiologic diuresis of extracellular fluid following transition to extrauterine life (Zangen et al., 2001) and from the passage of meconium.

Rodriguez et al. (2000) looked at 43 healthy term breastfed neonates over the first three days of life in Zaragosa University Clinic, Lozano, Spain. They weighed the babies and conducted bioelectrical impedance studies at the same time each day, calculating the percentage of total body water and the amount of body solids. Weight (the total body water and body solids) decreased progressively during the first three days of life. By day three, the average maximal weight loss was approximately 6% of the birth weight. The percentage of total body water, in other words, the hydration, actually increased slightly because there was a greater loss of body solids (the stool that was passed) than the loss of total body water.

Another study (Marchini & Stock, 1997) from Baby Friendly-certified Karolinska Hospital in Stockholm, Sweden, where no supplements were given unless weight loss exceeded 10% of birth weight, looked at 139 term healthy infants over the first three days of life. The babies who lost greater than 10% of their birth weight were fed more frequently than the cohort that lost less than 10% of birth weight. The serum sodium, serum osmolality, and plasma vasopressin remained the same over the three days, except for the group that lost greater than 10% of birth weight (Table 1.5). The hematocrit did not change. The authors concluded that in exclusively breastfed infants, maximal weight reduction averages about 6% of birthweight and occurs in the first one to two days. Most exclusively breastfed infants started to regain weight by the time they were three days old. The authors hypothesized that the decrease in feeding interval in the group that lost greater than 10% of birth weight was possibly because the babies are hungrier and thirstier, wanting to nurse more frequently.

Thirst and Vasopressin Secretion Counteract Dehydration in Newborn Infants						
Age (days)	Feeding Int (Hrs)	% B Wt Decrease	Serum Na	Serum Osmolality	Plasma Vasopressin	Hct
0	5	3.2	142	296	3.2	57
1	4.4	5.7	145	302	3.4	56
2	3.3	5.7	144	302	2.5	56
3	3.6	4.3	144	300	2.3	57
(2·5)*	2.4	11.8	150	312	6.9	55
* Group with > 10% weight loss						

Table 1.5. Weight Loss, Serum Sodium, and Plasma Vasopressin. Source: Marchini & Stock, J Pediatr 1997; 130(5):736-739. Reproduced with permission from Elsevier.

A retrospective observational cohort study of 937 consecutive term newborns of birthweight ≥ 2500 g during the first two to three weeks of life was done in a maternity service providing geographically defined community-based newborn follow up (MacDonald, Ross, Grant, & Yound, 2003). Of these infants, 45% were breastfed, 42% were formula fed, and 13% were breast and formula fed. The median weight loss, timing of loss, and days to regain birth weight are in Table 1.6. As expected, the artificially fed infants lost less weight and regained birth weight sooner. Remember, the breastfed infant is the norm, and insufficient weight loss in the newborn period may have later impact on obesity (Stettler et al., 2005)!

Neonatal weight loss in breast and formula fed infants			
	Breastfeeding	Formula feeding	Mixed
Maximal weight loss (%)	6.6	3.5	5.9
Timing of weight loss (days)	2.7	2.7	2.5
Regain birth weight (days)	8.3	6.5	7.9

Table 1.6. Neonatal Weight Loss in Breast-, Formula-, and Mixed-Fed Infants. Data Source: McDonald et al, Arch Dis Child Fetal Neonatal Ed 2003; 88(6): F472-476).

A more recent study looked at factors associated with in-hospital weight loss (Table 1.7; Martens & Romphf, 2007). In this study, mixed fed infants lost as much weight as their exclusively breastfed counterparts, but spent more days in the hospital, possibly because of a higher rate of cesarean section.

Factors Associated with Newborn In-Hospital Weight Loss			
Variable (P<0.05)	Exclusively breastfed (n=428)	Partially breastfed (n=275)	Completely formula fed (n=108)
Weight loss, % ± SD	5.49 ± 2.60	5.52 ± 3.02	2.43 ± 2.12
Days in hospital ± SD	2.13 ± 0.85	2.95 ± 1.33	2.53 ± 1.82
Multipara, %	66.6	58.8	70.4
Cesarean section, %	8.6	22.2	15.6
Epidural, %	21.5	36.4	22.0

Table 1.7. Factors Associated with Newborn In-Hospital Weight Loss. Source: Adapted from Martens and Romphf, JHL, 2007;23(3):233-241. Used with permission from Sage.

Many other studies have sought to ascertain the "normal" pattern of weight loss and gain for breastfed infants (Table 1.8). Crossland, Richmond, Hudson, Smith, and Abu-Harb (2008) weighed 111 term exclusively breastfed and 142 artificially-fed infants daily for the first two weeks of life. The mean maximal weight loss in the exclusively breastfed infants was 6.4% (CI 5.5–7.3%), with 54% of infants taking more than eight days to regain birthweight (Figure 1.2). In 2008 Noel-Weiss, Courant, and Woodend published a meta-analysis of 11 studies. The mean maximum weight loss was 5.7 to 6.6%, with standard deviations of approximately 2% and timing of two to three days. The majority of infants regained birthweight within the first two weeks of life. However, the methods used to report weight loss were inconsistent. More research is needed to understand the causes of neonatal weight loss, as well as the implications for morbidity and mortality.

Additional Weight Loss Studies		
Authors, Date	**Sample**	**Weight Loss**
Maisels, et al. (1988)	186 BF infants in well baby nursery	6.86% (SD 2.97%)
Yamauchi & Yamanouchi (1990)	112 BF non-rooming in & 92 BF rooming in, SVD, > 37 wk, Glu water & formula supplements	5.5% (SD 1.5%) not RI 6.4% (SD 1.9%) RI
Salariya & Robertson (1993)	63 breastfed ≥ 37 wks, rooming-in, may have supplementary feeds	6.63% (SD 2.5%)
Maisels et al (1994)	275 BF infants ≥ 36 wks, randomly assigned to frequent or on demand feed	5.5% frequent feeding 4.8% on demand feeding
Marchini, Fried, et al. (1998)	120 exclusively BF ≥ 37 wks, divided into 4 groups of 30 each	3.2 % at 16 hr age 6.0% on day 1; 6.4% on day 2; 5.7% on day 3
Hall, Simon, Smith (2000)	43 BF, ≥ 38 wks, modified demand feeding with Glu offered after each feeding	5.3% (SD 3.9%) at day 3
Hintz et al (2001)	64 exclusively BF ≥ 37 wks, C/S	7.0% (SD 2.4%) at day 3
Dewey et al. (2003)	280 BF, ≥ 37 wks, < 2 oz supplementation	5.5% (SD 3.8%) on day 3
Davanzo et al. (2012)	1003 BF and formula-fed infants, weight loss protocol	6.7% (SD 2.2%)

Table 1.8. Additional Weight Loss Studies

Change in Body Weight Based on Birthweight

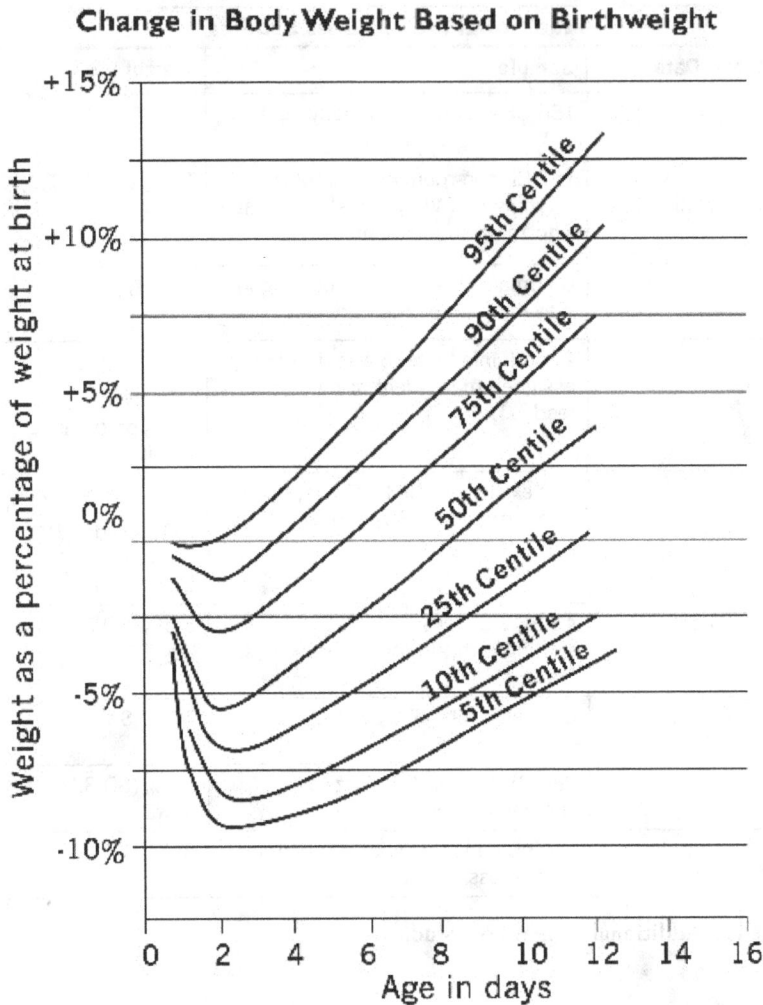

Figure 1.2. Change in Body Weight Based on Birthweight. Source: Crossland et al. Acta Paediatrica 2008; 97(4):425-429. Reproduced with permission from John Wiley and Sons.

Three more recent studies deserve discussion. Mulder, Johnson, and Baker (2010) followed a convenience sample of 53 breastfeeding women. The mean maximal infant weight loss was 5.69%. Twenty-one percent lost greater than or equal to 7% of birthweight, and those infants had more total voids and greater breastfeeding frequency than infants who lost less than 7% of birthweight. This suggested the excess weight loss might have been due to physiologic diuresis, unrelated to breastfeeding behaviors. Flaherman, Bokser, and Newman (2010) followed 1,049 exclusively breastfed term infants and found that although the mean in-hospital weight nadir was 6.0 ± 2.6%, those infants who lost ≥ 4.5% of birth weight at less than 24 hours had a greater risk of in-hospital loss of ≥ 10% (AOR 3.57). A possible explanation for this excess early weight loss is an excess of maternal fluids during labor (Chantry, Nommsen-Rivers, Peerson, Cohen, & Dewey, 2011).

Knowing "normal" is important for anticipatory guidance, appropriate treatment of patients, and avoiding both short- and long-term harm. However, as with ANY aspect of medicine, "normal" depends upon wide physiologic variation, cultural expectations, caregiver education and experience, and social changes over time. In the U.S., we would have less trouble with breastfeeding if all women had mL marks on their breasts! In the meantime, the golden rule is "what goes in must come out." Adequate intake can be judged by many factors:

- A maximal weight loss of < 8% by day three to four.

    ◊ Some weight stabilization or gain as the milk supply increases on day four to five.

    ◊ Regaining birthweight by day 10–14.

- Yellow, seedy, curdy cottage cheese and mustard stools by day five.

- Feeding every two to three hours on average (eight to 12 times per 24 hours) in the first few weeks, and acting satisfied.

- Normal tone and activity.

- Jaundice stable or decreasing.

One study found the most efficient predictor of breastfeeding *inadequacy* to be less than four soiled diapers on day four, plus the onset of increasing milk supply (lactogenesis II or secretory activation) at greater than 72 hours (Nommsen-Rivers, Heinig, Cohen, & Dewey, 2008), although the low specificity might lead to many false positives. Anticipatory guidance should include:

- Colostrum vs. mature milk (volume, appearance, purpose)

- Stool progression (meconium, green, yellow)

- Growth/appetite spurts (increased nursing and decreased stools)

- Nursing frequency and duration (wide variation; infant, not clock directed)

- Signs of let-down (variation, intensity, timing)

Chapter 2. Hypoglycemia

Glucose Homeostasis

Healthy, full-term infants are programmed to make the transition from their intrauterine constant flow of nutrients to their extrauterine intermittent nutrient intake, without the need for metabolic monitoring or interference with the natural breastfeeding process. Homeostatic mechanisms ensure adequate energy substrate is provided to the brain and other organs, even when feedings are delayed. The normal pattern of early, frequent, and exclusive breastfeeding meets the needs of healthy full-term infants (Adamkin, 2011; Rozance & Hay, 2010; Wight, 2006; Wight, Marinelli, & ABM Protocol Committee, 2006; Williams, 1997). In the past infants were not fed for four to 12 hours for "stabilization." However, at present, far too many infants are given supplements based on an arbitrary glucose value, without an understanding of normal transitional glucose physiology. In addition, many late preterm (34 to 36 6/7weeks) infants are remaining with their mothers and need special attention to prevent hypoglycemia, jaundice, and overall poor nutritional intake.

Throughout gestation the fetus receives its entire supply of glucose (70% of its energy needs) from the maternal circulation by facilitated diffusion via the placenta, with fetal plasma glucose levels 70–80% of maternal venous plasma levels (Williams, 1997). Glucose utilization by the fetus is approximately 4–6 mg/kg/minute, with amino acids and lactate as additional energy sources (Rozance & Hay, 2010). Although present, the enzyme activity necessary for gluconeogenesis (the production of glucose from other substrates) is minimal in the fetus, as there is no need for glucose production. However, an important sequence of integrated metabolic adaptations occurs at birth, allowing the newborn to produce glucose and regulate its own metabolic homeostatic processes (Sperling & Menon, 2004). At birth the infant must supply its glucose needs of approximately 5–8 mg/kg/min (70% utilized by the brain) through a balance of exogenous sources (breastmilk) and endogenous glucose production through gluconeogenesis, glycogenolysis (production of glucose through breakdown of glycogen in the liver), and ketogenesis (production of ketones as an alternate brain fuel), provided adequate substrates are available (Eidelman, 2001; Sperling & Menon, 2004). Maintenance of glucose homeostasis depends on the balance between hepatic glucose output and peripheral glucose utilization (Figure 2.1).

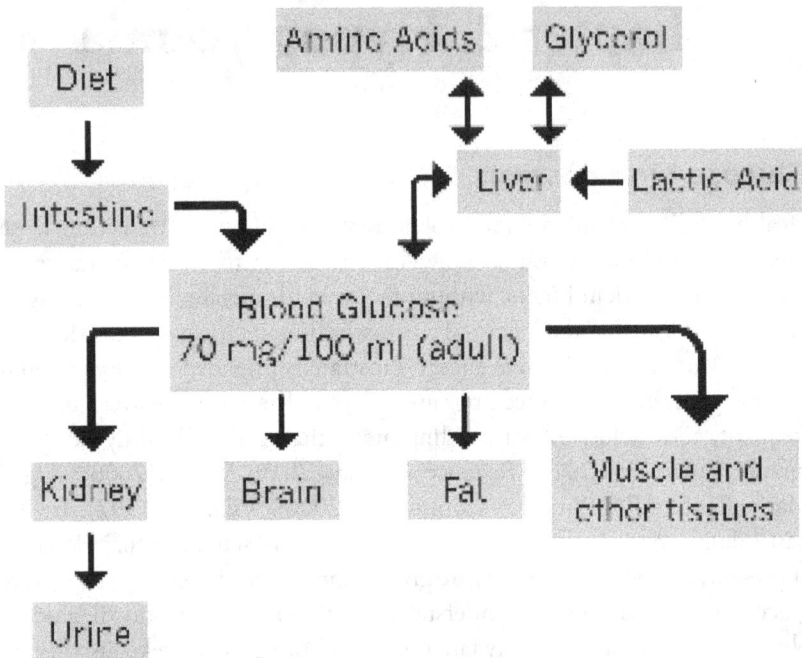

Figure 2.1. Blood Glucose Homeostasis

Within minutes of the cutting of the umbilical cord, there is a three-to five-fold surge in glucagon and catecholamines, which initiate glycogen breakdown. High endogenous growth hormone and cortisol facilitate the onset of gluconeogenesis within several hours, and insulin secretion is blunted so that serum concentrations of insulin fall (Sperling & Menon, 2004). The processes that ensure the availability of glucose and other fuels are collectively described as *counter-regulation*, and are activated primarily by glucagon and adrenalin (Sperling & Menon, 2004).

The term *hypoglycemia* refers to a low blood glucose concentration. Neonatal hypoglycemia is not a medical condition in itself, but a feature of another illness or a failure to adapt from the fetal state of continuous transplacental glucose consumption to the extrauterine pattern of intermittent nutrient supply (Williams, 1997). Transient hypoglycemia in the immediate newborn period is ubiquitous among mammals and is a normal physiologic function that is essential for activating glucose production in the neonate. In healthy term human infants, even if early enteral feeding is withheld, this phenomenon is self-limited, as glucose levels spontaneously rise within two to three hours (Cornblath & Reisner, 1965; Hawdon, Ward Platt, & Aynsley-Green, 1992; Srinivasan, Pildes, Cattamanchi, Voora, & Lilien, 1986). This early self-limited period of hypoglycemia cannot be considered pathological, and there is little practical value in measuring the blood glucose concentrations of asymptomatic babies in the first two hours after birth (Eidelman, 2001; Hawdon, Ward Platt, & Aynsley-Green, 1994; Wight et al., 2006; Williams, 1997). Furthermore, even in those situations where low blood glucose concentrations develop secondary to prolonged intervals (> 8 hours) between breastfeedings (Hawdon et al., 1992), there is a marked ketogenic response which provides glucose-sparing fuel to the brain (Edmond, Auestad, Robbins, & Bergstrom, 1985; Hawdon et al., 1992; Lucas, Boyes, Bloom, & Aynsley-Green, 1981; Yager, Heitjan, Towfighi, & Vannucci, 1992). The neonatal brain has an enhanced capability to utilize ketone bodies relative to infants (four-fold) and adults (40-fold; Mehta, 1994).

Hawdon et al. (1992) and others have studied this pattern of metabolic adaptation (Heck & Erenberg, 1987; Swenne, Ewald, Gustafsson, Sandberg, & Ostenson, 1994). Breastfed term infants have lower blood glucose (Durand et al., 1997; Hawdon et al., 1992; Heck & Erenberg, 1987; Swenne et al., 1994) and higher ketone bodies (Hawdon et al., 1992) than formula-fed infants. Breastfed infants up to one week old had a significantly lower mean blood glucose concentration (range 1.5–5.3 mmol/L [27–95 mg/dL] and mean 3.6 mmol/L [58 mg/dL]) than formula-fed infants of the same age (range 2.5–6.2 mmol/L [45–111 mg/dL] and mean 4.0 mmol/L [72 mg/dL]; Hawdon et al., 1992). Those infants who lost the most weight postnatally had the highest ketone body concentration, which suggests that the provision of alternate fuels constitutes a normal adaptive response to transiently low nutrient intake during the establishment of breastfeeding (Cornblath et al., 2000; Hawdon et al., 1992). As the optimally breastfed infant's lower blood glucose is the physiologic norm, it has been suggested that breastfed infants may well tolerate lower plasma glucose levels without any significant clinical manifestations or sequellae, assuming adaptive metabolic response systems are functioning normally.

Definitions of Hypoglycemia

The definition of hypoglycemia in the newborn infant has remained controversial because of a lack of significant correlation between plasma glucose concentration, clinical symptoms, and long-term sequelae (Boluyt, van Kempen, & Offringa, 2006; Cornblath et al., 2000; Kalhan & Peter-Wohl, 2000; Sinclair, 1997). There have been four main approaches to the definition of hypoglycemia (Cornblath et al., 2000; Williams, 1997):

1. Epidemiological/statistical approach based on measured range of glucose values

2. Clinical manifestations

3. Acute changes in metabolic/endocrine responses and neurologic function

4. Long-term neurologic outcome

Epidemiologic Approach. "Normal" blood glucose results vary enormously with the source of the blood sample, the assay method, and whether blood or plasma glucose concentration is determined. Plasma or serum glucose concentrations are 10–15% higher than in whole blood (Cornblath & Schwartz, 1991). In addition, feeding schedules have a prominent effect on blood glucose concentrations, but have changed a great deal since early studies (Williams, 1997). Even now, they vary from hospital to hospital. The healthy, term breastfed infant represents the biological norm, yet, until recently, very few breastfed infants had been studied.

Breastfed, formula-fed, and mixed-fed infants follow the same pattern of glucose values, with an initial fall in glucose over the first one to two hours, followed by a gradual rise in glucose over the next 96 hours, whether fed or not (Figure 2.2).

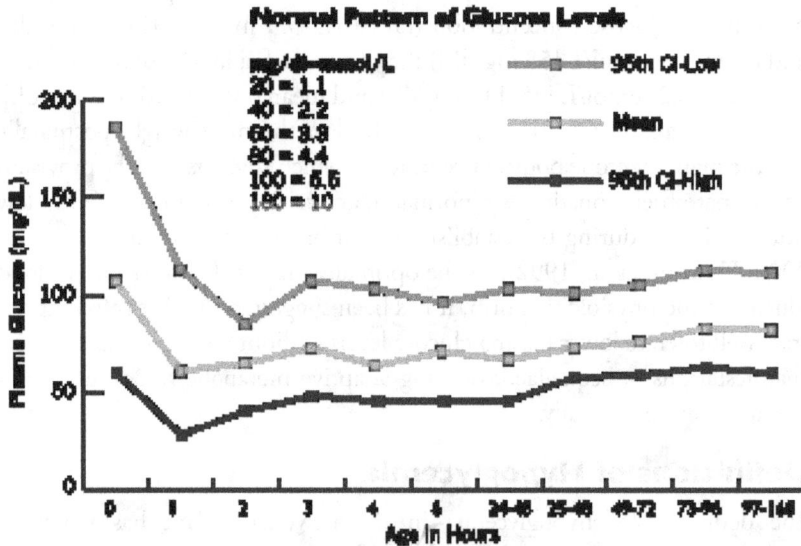

Figure 2.2. **Normal Pattern of Glucose Levels. Source:** Srinivasan G, Pildes RS, Cattamanchi G, et al. Plasma glucose values in normal neonates: A new look. J Pediatr 1986; 109(1):114-117. Reproduced with permission from Elsevier.

Although helpful, the findings of the epidemiologic approach have been inaccurately used to define the cutoff between normoglycemia and hypoglycemia, rather than recognizing that hypoglycemia reflects a continuum of biologic abnormalities, ranging from mild to severe (Cornblath et al., 2000).

The incidence of "hypoglycemia" varies with the definition (Sexson, 1984). Many authors have suggested numerical definitions of hypoglycemia, usually between 30–50 mg/dL (1.7 – 2.8 mmol/L) and varying by postnatal age (Alkalay, Klein, Nagel, & Sola, 2001; Alkalay et al., 2006; Cole & Peevy, 1994; Heck & Erenberg, 1987; Kalhan & Peter-Wohl, 2000; Koh, Eyre, & Aynsley-Green, 1988; Schwartz, 1997; Sexson, 1984; Srinivasan et al., 1986; Stanley & Baker, 1999; Williams, 1997). Cornblath et al. (2000) summarized the problem well: "Significant hypoglycemia is not and can not be defined as a single number that can be applied universally to every individual patient. Rather, it is characterized by a value(s) that is unique to each individual and varies with both their state of physiologic maturity and the influence of pathology." Instead of specifying a number to represent hypoglycemia, Cornblath and colleagues (Cornblath et al., 2000; Cornblath & Ichord, 2000) suggest "operational thresholds" as defined by Table 2.1. These "operational thresholds" represent values which require some response, either by further assessment and/or treatment. *They do not represent either normal or abnormal values.*

Operational Threshold for Plasma Glucose	
Intervention	< 36 mg/dL (2.0 mmol/L)
IV Glucose	< 20-25 mg/dL (1.1-1.4 mmol/L)
Preterm infants	same as term
Infants on TPN	> 45 mg/dL (2.5 mmol/L)
Therapeutic Objective	
Transient hypoglycemia	> 45 mg/dL (2.5 mmol/L)
Profound/persistent hypoglycemia	> 60 mg/dL (3.3 mmol/L)
Operational Thresholds by Age After Birth	
1st 24 hrs:	
Healthy term or preterm 34-37 weeks, formula-fed:	< 30-35 mg/dL (1.7-2.0 mmol/L)
Sick, LBW, preterm < 34 wks:	< 45-50 mg/dL (2.5-2.8 mmol/L)
> 24 hrs:	< 40-50 mg/dL (2.2-2.8 mmol/L)
Any age:	20-25 mg/dL (1.1-1.4 mmol/L)

Table 2.1. Operational Thresholds for Plasma Glucose. Source: Modified from: Cornblath, M., Hawdon, J. M., Williams, A. F., Aynsley-Green, A., Ward-Platt, M. P., Schwartz, R., et al. (2000). Controversies regarding definition of neonatal hypoglycemia: suggested operational thresholds. Pediatrics, 105(5), 1141-1145 and Cornblath, M., & Ichord, R. (2000). Hypoglycemia in the neonate. Semin Perinatol, 24(2), 136-149.

A meta-analysis (studies published 1986–1994) of plasma glucose levels in full-term normal newborns who were mostly mixed fed (formula and breastfeeding) or formula-fed, presented recommended low thresholds for plasma glucose based on hours after birth (Table 2.2). They specifically noted that given the lower plasma glucose levels in normal breastfed infants, the low thresholds for exclusively breastfed infants might even be lower (Alkalay et al., 2006).

Recommended Low Thresholds: Plasma Glucose Level	
Hour after Birth	≤ 5th percentile PGL·mg/dL (mmol/L)
1·2 (nadir)	28 (1.6)
3·47	40 (2.2)
48·72	48 (2.7)

Table 2.2. Recommended Low Thresholds for Plasma Glucose Levels
Source: Adapted from Alkalay et al. Am J Perinatol, 23(2): 115-119

Clinical Manifestations of Hypoglycemia Approach. The clinical manifestations of hypoglycemia are *non-specific*, occurring with a variety of other neonatal problems. Even in the presence of an arbitrary low glucose level, the physician must assess the general status of the infant by observation and physical exam to rule out other disease entities and processes that may need additional laboratory evaluation and treatment. Some common clinical signs are listed in Table 2.3. A diagnosis of hypoglycemia also requires that symptoms abate after normoglycemia is restored.

Clinical Manifestations of Possible Hypoglycemia

Irritability, tremors, jitteriness

Exaggerated Moro reflex

High·pitched cry

Seizures or myoclonic jerks

Lethargy, listlessness, limpness, hyoptonia

Coma

Cyanosis

Apnea or irregular breathing

Tachypnea

Hypothermia

Vasomotor instability

Poor suck or refusal to feed

Table 2.3. Clinical Manifestations of Possible Hypoglycemia

Acute Physiologic Changes Approach. Neurophysiologic monitoring, including electroencephalography (EEG), visual evoked potentials (VEP), and brainstem auditory evoked responses (BAER), have failed to define a safe blood glucose concentration or a threshold for neurologic damage (Eidelman, 2001). Koh, Aynsley-Green, Tarbit, and Eyre (1988) reported BAER abnormalities only when blood glucose fell below 2.6 mmol/L (47 mg/dL). Unfortunately, only five of their 17 patients were less than four days old, only one was symptomatic, and the symptoms did not correlate with the lowest blood glucose level. Kinnala et al. (1999) found four times the number of head MRI and ultrasound abnormalities in 18 *symptomatic* full-term infants than 19 normoglycemic controls. Most lesions were absent by two months of age, and only one infant appeared neurologically affected.

Evidence from tissue culture and animal models indicate that the neural damage attributed to hypoglycemia is not simply a matter of inadequate energy stores, but rather a result of accumulation of toxic substances, such as aspartic acid (Eidelman, 2001) and glutamate (McGowan, 1999). Because this process requires time (hours to days), clinicians can be reassured that transient, single, brief periods of hypoglycemia are unlikely to cause permanent neurologic damage (American Academy of Pediatrics Committee on Fetus and Newborn, 1993; Cornblath & Ichord, 2000; Eidelman, 2001; Hawdon, 1999; McGowan, 1999).

Long-Term Neurologic Outcome Approach. The data correlating neonatal hypoglycemia with long-term neurologic outcome are limited because of lack of suitable non-hypoglycemic controls, failure to consider other pathology, and the small number of asymptomatic infants followed (Boluyt et al., 2006; Cornblath et al., 2000; Sinclair, 1997). Animal studies suggest that the immature brain is incredibly resistant (via many different mechanisms) to damage from even profound hypoglycemia (Vannucci & Vannucci, 2001). Koivisto, Blanco-Sequeiros, and Krause (1972) found no difference in neurologic outcome between asymptomatic hypoglycemic infants and euglycemic control infants, with 94% and 95% of each group normal on one to four year follow-up. There was a significant increase in neurologic abnormalities (12%) in *symptomatic* (tremor, cyanosis, paleness, limpness, irritability, apathy, or tachypnea, which disappeared during treatment with glucose) hypoglycemic infants, and 50% incidence of neurologic abnormalities when seizures were present. The estimated duration of hypoglycemia was 37 hours in the asymptomatic hypoglycemic infants, 49 hours in the symptomatic/non-seizure group, and 105 hours in the seizure group. The follow-up evaluation included a physical exam, anthropometry, neurologic and developmental assessments, as well as an ophthalmologic exam. Interestingly, this study was done in Finland during 1967–1970, at a time when infants were fed 5% "saccharose" for 24 hours prior to initiating breastfeeding.

More recently, Brand, Molenaar, Kaaijk, and Wierenga (2005) studied hypoglycemia (defined as < 2.2 mmol/L [<40 mg/dL] one hour after birth or < 2.5 mmol/L [<45 mg/dL] thereafter) in term LGA infants born to non-diabetic mothers. Screening was done at one, three, and five hours after birth and continued if the glucose was low. Intravenous glucose was started if the glucose was < 1.5–2.0 mmol/L (27–36 mg/dL) or symptoms were present. There were no significant differences between the hypoglycemic and control groups at their four-year follow-up. Unfortunately, the type of feeding was not disclosed, and only 64% of the original population completed the assessment at four years.

A systematic review of cohort studies on subsequent neurologic development after episodes of hypoglycemia in the first week of life found that major clinical and methodologic heterogeneity of available studies precluded any true meta-analysis (Boluyt et al., 2006). None of the studies provided a valid estimate of the effect of neonatal hypoglycemia on neurodevelopment. Another systematic review attempted to determine which low glucose concentrations, their duration, and their association with clinical signs might indicate potential long-term neurologic injury (Table 2.4; Rozance & Hay, 2006). The effect of any set of guidelines to manage glucose concentrations in neonates on preventing long-term complications of "hypoglycemia" (however defined) has never been tested by a large, randomized, controlled trial.

Conditions that should be present before considering that long term neurological impairment might be related to neonatal hypoglycemia:

1. Blood or plasma glucose concentrations below 1 mmol/ (18 mg/dl). Such values definitely are abnormal; although if transient, there is no study in the literature confirming that they lead to permanent neurological injury.

2. Persistence of such severely low glucose concentrations for prolonged periods (hours, probably >2–3 h, rather than minutes, although there is no study in human neonates that defines this period).

3. Early mild-to-moderate clinical signs (primarily those of increased adrenalin [epinephrine] activity), such as alternating CNS signs of jitteriness/tremulousness vs. stupor/lethargy or even a brief convulsion, that diminish or disappear with effective treatment that promptly restores the glucose concentration to the statistically normal range (>45 mg/dl).

4. More serious clinical signs that are prolonged (many hours or longer), including coma, seizures, respiratory depression and/ or apnea with cyanosis, hypotonia or limpness, high-pitched cry, hypothermia, and poor feeding after initially feeding well; these are more refractory to short-term treatment.

5. Concurrence of associated conditions, particularly persistent excessive insulin secretion and hyperinsulinemia with repeated episodes of acute, severe hypoglycemia with seizures and/or coma (although sub-clinical, often severe, hypoglycemic episodes occur in these conditions and might be just as injurious).

Table 2.4. Conditions for Hypoglycemia Neurologic Impairment Causality
Source: Adapted from Rozance and Hay, Biol Neonate 2006; 90(2):74-86).

Dr. Hawdon (1999) summarized it well: "Evidence from studies of humans and other animals suggests that cortical damage and long-term sequelae occur after prolonged hypoglycemia sufficiently severe to cause neurological signs." In the absence of definitive data regarding a "safe" blood glucose concentration in any given population, the "operational threshold" approach suggested by Cornblath (Cornblath et al., 2000; Cornblath & Ichord, 2000) and Alkalay (Alkalay et al., 2006) seems most appropriate.

Several assessment and treatment algorithms have been suggested. Rozance and Hay (2006) produced an algorithm, but were careful to note that the levels chosen were arbitrary and not "normal" or "hypoglycemic" (Figure 2.3). Jain et al. (2010) suggested an algorithm defining hypoglycemia as a blood glucose level less than 40 mg/dL (plasma glucose less than 45 mg/dL) based on a workshop report by Hay, Raju, Higgins, Kalhan, & Devaskar (2009). Most recently, the American Academy of Pediatrics Committee on Fetus and Newborn published a clinical report as a practical guide for screening and subsequent management of neonatal hypoglycemia (Figure 2.4; Adamkin, 2011).

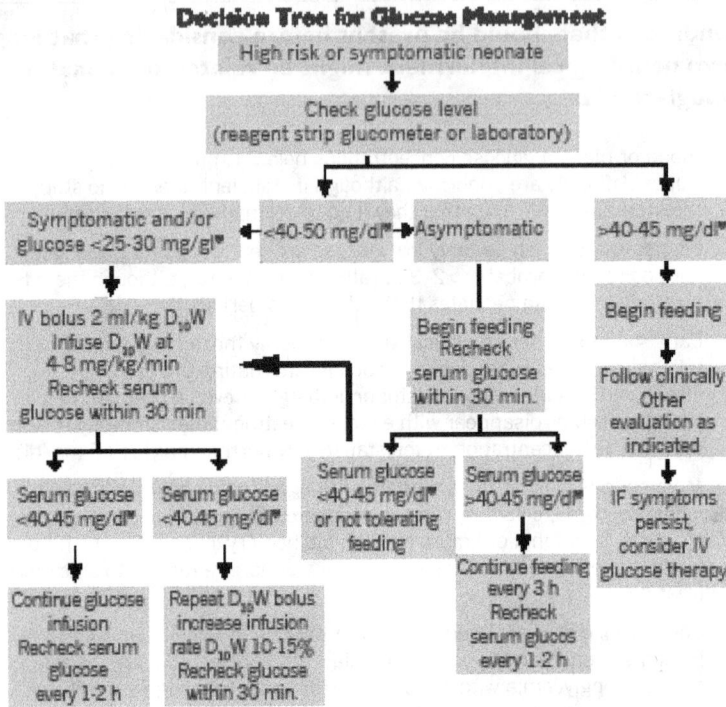

Decision Tree for Glucose Management

High risk or symptomatic neonate

Check glucose level
(reagent strip glucometer or laboratory)

Symptomatic and/or glucose <25-30 mg/gl▪ ◄— <40-50 mg/dl▪ —► Asymptomatic   >40-45 mg/dl▪

IV bolus 2 ml/kg D$_{10}$W
Infuse D$_{10}$W at
4-8 mg/kg/min
Recheck serum
glucose within 30 min

Begin feeding
Recheck
serum glucose
within 30 min.

Begin feeding

Follow clinically
Other
evaluation as
indicated

Serum glucose <40-45 mg/dl▪   Serum glucose <40-45 mg/dl▪

Serum glucose <40-45 mg/dl▪ or not tolerating feeding   Serum glucose >40-45 mg/dl▪

IF symptoms
persist,
consider IV
glucose therapy

Continue glucose infusion
Recheck serum glucose every 1-2 h

Repeat D$_{10}$W bolus increase infusion rate D$_{10}$W 10-15%
Recheck glucose within 30 min.

Continue feeding every 3 h
Recheck
serum glucos
every 1-2 h

Figure 2.3. Decision Tree for Glucose Management (Rozance & Hay, 2006).
Source: Rozance, P. J., & Hay, W. W. (2006). Hypoglycemia in newborn infants: Features associated with adverse outcomes. Biol Neonate, 90(2), 74-86. Used with permission from Karger.

Screening and management of Postnatal Glucose Homeostasis in Late Pre-term and Term SGA, IDM/LGA Infants [(LPT) Infants 34-36 weeks and SGA (screen 0-24 hrs); IDM and LGA≥34 weeks (screen 0-12 hrs)]			
Symptomatic and <40 mg/dL —> IV Glucose			
ASYMPTOMATIC			
Birth to 4 hours of age		4-24 hours of age	
INITIAL FEED WITHIN 1 hour Screen glucose 30 minutes after 1st feed		Continue feeds q 2-3 hours Screen glucose prior to each feed	
Initial screen <25 mg/dL		Screen <35 mg/dL	
Feed and check in 1 hour		Feed and check in 1 hour	
<25 mg/dL ↓ ∨ IV glucose*	24-40 mg/dL ↓ ∨ Refeed/IV glucose* as needed	<35 mg/dL ↓ ∨ IV glucose*	35-45 mg/dL ↓ ∨ Refeed/IV glucose* as needed
Target glucose screen ≥45 mg/dL prior to routine feeds *glucose dose = 200 mg/kg (dextrose 10% at 2 mL/kg) and/or IV infusion at 5-8 mg/kg per min (80-100 mL/kg per d). Achieve plasma gluose level of 40-50 mg/dL.			
Symptoms of hypoglycemia include: Irritability, tremors, jitteriness, exaggerated Moro reflex, high-pitched cry, seizures, lethargy, floppiness, cyanosis, apnea, poorfeeding.			
Screening for and management of postnatal glucose homeostasis in late-preterm (LPT 34-36 weeks) and term small-for-gestational age (SGA) infants and infants who were born to mothers with diabetes (IDM)/large-for-gestational age (LGA) infants. LPT and SGA (screen 0-24 hours), IDM and LGA ≥34 weeks (screen 0-12 hours). IV indicates intravenous.			

Figure 2.4. AAP Clinical Report – Glucose Algorithm (Adamkin, 2011).
Source: Adamkin, Pediatrics 2011; 127(3):575-579. Used with permission from AAP.

Assessment of Glucose Levels

Bedside glucose testing strips are inexpensive and practical, but are not reliable, with significant variance from true blood glucose levels (Alkalay et al., 2001; Hawdon, Platt, & Aynsley-Green, 1993; Ho, Yeung, & Young, 2004). Studies comparing different reagent strips have estimated that as many as 20% of truly normoglycemic infants are falsely labeled as hypoglycemic, leading to unnecessary laboratory tests and treatment (Eidelman, 2001). A recent study evaluated readily available "point-of-care" glucose measuring devices and concluded that none of the five glucometers was satisfactory as the sole measuring device (Ho et al., 2004). Newer bedside glucose systems simplify procedures, but appropriate test strip storage, handling, and adherence to expiration dates are still essential to prevent error (Sirkin, Jalloh, & Lee, 2002).

Although a possible improvement over reagent strips, even newer point-of-care glucose electrode (YSI) and cuvette-based glucose oxidation optical methods (HemoCue) do not have the reliability of laboratory measurement (Dahlberg & Whitelaw, 1997; Ellis et al., 1996; Sharief & Hussein, 1997; Williams, 1997). Bedside glucose tests may be utilized for screening, but laboratory levels must confirm results before a diagnosis of hypoglycemia can be made, especially in asymptomatic infants (Adamkin, 2011; American Academy of Pediatrics Committee on Fetus and Newborn, 1993; Cornblath & Schwartz, 1991; Hawdon et al., 1993; Hay et al., 2009; Williams, 1997).

Risk Factors for Hypoglycemia

Neonates at increased risk for developing neonatal hypoglycemia should be routinely monitored for blood glucose levels irrespective of the mode of feeding. These at-risk infants should be screened *before* any symptoms manifest. Neonates at risk fall into two main categories (Cornblath & Ichord, 2000):

1. Excess utilization of glucose, which includes the hyperinsulinemic states

2. Inadequate production or substrate delivery

Table 2.5 lists maternal and infant conditions that increase the risk of hypoglycemia in the neonate (Cornblath et al., 2000; Cornblath & Ichord, 2000; Cowett & Loughead, 2002; de Lonlay, Giurgea, Touati, & Saudubray, 2004; Eidelman, 2001; Sunehag & Haymond, 2002).

Conditions Indicating Risk of Neonatal Hypoglycemia

Maternal Conditions:

Diabetes or abnormal glucose tolerance test result

Hypertensive disorders of pregnancy

Maternal beta-blocker medication

Previous macrosomic infants

Maternal beta-agonist tocolytics

Maternal oral hypoglycemic agents

Neonatal Conditions:

Preterm birth

Intrauterine growth restriction (IUGR/SGA); < 10th percentile for weight

Large for gestational age (LGA); >90th percentile for weight*

Discordant twin; weight 10% < larger twin

Low birth weight (<2500g)

After perinatal stress: severe acidosis or hypoxia-ischemia

Cold stress

Polycythemia (venous Hct > 70%)/ Hyperviscosity

Erythroblastosis fetalis

Beckwith-Wiedemann Syndrome

Microphallus or midline defect

Suspected infection

Respiratory distress

Known or suspected inborn errors of metabolism or endocrine disorders

Any infant admitted to the Neonatal Intensive Care Unit (NICU)

Iatrogenic administration of insulin

Infants displaying symptoms associated with hypoglycemia

* In unscreened populations where LGA may represent undiagnosed and untreated maternal diabetes.

Table 2.5. Risk Factors for Neonatal Hypoglycemia. Source: Adapted from Koh et al, Arch Dis Child 1988; 63(11):1353-1358 and Wight, Breastfeeding Med 2006; 1(4):253-262.

Breastfeeding-Supportive Management Recommendations

General. Glucose screening should be performed only on at-risk infants and those with clinical symptoms compatible with hypoglycemia. Routine monitoring of blood glucose in asymptomatic, term newborns is potentially harmful to the establishment of a healthy mother-infant relationship and successful breastfeeding patterns (AAP & ACOG, 2008; American Academy of Pediatrics Committee on Fetus and Newborn, 1993; American Academy of Pediatrics Section on Breastfeeding, 2012; Eidelman, 2001; Haninger & Farley, 2001; Hawdon et al., 1993; Hawdon et al., 1994; Nicholl, 2003; Wight et al., 2006; Williams, 1997). At-risk infants should be screened for hypoglycemia with a frequency and duration related to the specific risk factors of the individual infant (Eidelman, 2001). It is suggested that monitoring begin within 30–60 minutes for infants with suspected hyperinsulinemia, and no later than two hours of age for infants in other risk categories. Monitoring should continue until normal pre-prandial levels are consistently obtained. Bedside glucose screening tests must be confirmed by formal laboratory testing.

Early and exclusive breastfeeding meets the nutritional needs of healthy, term newborn infants. Healthy term infants do not develop symptomatic hypoglycemia simply as a result of underfeeding (American Academy of Pediatrics Section on Breastfeeding, 2012; Eidelman, 2001; Wight, 2006; Wight et al., 2006; Williams, 1997). Therefore, routine supplementation of healthy term infants with water, glucose water, or formula is unnecessary and may interfere with establishment of normal breastfeeding and normal metabolic compensatory mechanisms (American Academy of Pediatrics Section on Breastfeeding, 2012; Hawdon et al., 1992; Williams, A.F., 1997; Swenne et al., 1994; Wight, 2006). As with general breastfeeding recommendations, healthy term infants should initiate breastfeeding within 30–60 minutes of life and continue on demand, recognizing that crying is a very late sign of hunger (American Academy of Pediatrics Section on Breastfeeding, 2012; WHO/UNICEF, 1989). Feedings should be frequent, 10–12 times per 24 hours in the first few days after birth (American Academy of Pediatrics Section on Breastfeeding, 2012). Early breastfeeding is not precluded just because the infant meets the criteria for glucose monitoring. Initiation and establishment of breastfeeding is also facilitated by skin-to-skin contact of mother and infant. Such practices will maintain normal infant body temperature and reduce energy expenditure, while stimulating suckling and milk production (American Academy of Pediatrics Section on Breastfeeding, 2012; Durand et al., 1997).

Documented Hypoglycemia in an Asymptomatic Infant. As noted above, the asymptomatic "hypoglycemic" infant is at extremely low risk of long-term neurologic sequellae. Such an infant should continue breastfeeding (approximately every one to two hours) or feed 2–5 ml/kg of expressed breastmilk or substitute nutrition (pasteurized donor human milk, elemental formulas, partially hydrolyzed formulas, routine formulas). This volume is based on normal volumes of colostrum (Neville et al., 2001) and the average size of the infant's stomach in the first week post-partum (Scammon & Doyle, 1920). There is no research available delineating what amount of glucose or what volume of glucose-containing oral fluids is needed to raise serum glucose a certain amount in any population.

The blood glucose concentration should be rechecked before subsequent feedings until the value is acceptable and stable. If the neonate is unable to suck or feedings are not tolerated, avoid forced feedings (e.g., nasogastric tube) and begin intravenous therapy (see below). Such an infant is not normal and requires a careful examination and evaluation, in addition to more intensive therapy. If glucose remains low despite feedings, intravenous glucose therapy should be initiated and the intravenous rate adjusted by blood glucose concentration. Of course, breastfeeding may continue during IV glucose therapy if the infant is interested and will suckle. As with any medical therapy, clinical signs, physical examination, screening values, laboratory confirmation, treatment, and changes in clinical condition (i.e., response to treatment) should be carefully documented (Wight et al., 2006).

Symptomatic Hypoglycemic Infants. Infants with symptoms consistent with hypoglycemia (see Table 2.3 pg. 26) or infants with plasma glucose levels < 20–25 mg/dL (< 1.1–1.4 mmol/L) should have more aggressive therapy. Current neonatal texts suggest initiating intravenous glucose using a 2 ml/kg bolus of 10% glucose solution, followed by a continuous infusion of 6–8 mg/kg/minute (approximately 80–100 ml/kg/24 hours; Katz & Stanley, 2005; Lilien et al., 1980). Attempts to rely on oral or intragastric feeding to correct extreme (<20–25 mg/dL) or symptomatic hypoglycemia are inappropriate and may be dangerous if the infant aspirates the oral supplement. Such an infant is not normal and requires an immediate and careful examination and evaluation. To allow for minute-to-minute variations in blood glucose, the glucose concentration in symptomatic infants should be maintained > 45 mg/dL (> 2.5 mmol/L).

The intravenous rate should be adjusted by blood glucose concentration, and frequent breastfeeding should be encouraged after the relief of symptoms. As feedings are initiated and the IV is weaned, glucose concentrations should be monitored before feedings until values are stabilized off intravenous fluids. Again, clinical signs, physical examination, screening values, laboratory confirmation, treatment, and changes in clinical condition (i.e., response to treatment) should be carefully documented (Wight et al., 2006).

Supporting the Mother

Having an infant thought to be normal and healthy develop hypoglycemia is concerning to the mother and family, and may jeopardize breastfeeding. Mothers should be reassured that there is nothing wrong with their milk, and that supplementation is usually temporary. Having the mother hand-express or pump milk that is then fed to her infant can overcome feelings of maternal inadequacy, as well as help establish a full milk supply (Wight et al., 2006). In order to protect the mother's milk supply, it is important to provide stimulation to the breasts by manual or mechanical expression with appropriate frequency (eight times in 24 hours) until her baby is latching and suckling well. Keeping the infant at breast or returning the infant to the breast as soon as possible is important. Skin-to-skin care is easily done with an IV and may soften the trauma of intervention, while providing physiologic thermoregulation, contributing to metabolic homeostasis.

Hypoglycemia Summary

Healthy full-term infants are programmed to make the transition from their intrauterine constant flow of nutrients to their extra-uterine intermittent nutrient intake without the need for metabolic monitoring or interference with the natural breastfeeding process. Homeostatic mechanisms ensure adequate energy substrate is provided to the brain and other organs, even when feedings are delayed. The normal pattern of early, frequent, and exclusive breastfeeding meets the needs of healthy full-term infants. Routine screening or supplementation are not necessary and may harm the normal establishment of breastfeeding. Screening should be restricted to AT RISK and symptomatic infants. Symptomatic infants need immediate assessment and intravenous glucose therapy, not forced feedings.

The neurological impact of a given plasma glucose concentration in a given infant is dependent on multiple factors. No systematic studies have been done to demonstrate the risks or benefits of using a specific blood glucose concentration as a threshold for intervention in neonatal hypoglycemia for any group of infants. Therefore, using any specific blood glucose concentration to define neonatal hypoglycemia is without rigorous scientific justification. The key to preventing complications from glucose deficiency is to focus less on numerical values of glucose concentration and more on identifying infants at risk, promoting early and frequent feedings, measuring glucose concentrations as appropriate, and treating promptly when glucose deficiency is severe and symptomatic.

Chapter 3. Neonatal Jaundice

Introduction

Neonatal jaundice is a very common problem, both in the hospital and after discharge. It is one of the most common reasons for hospital readmission. As breastfeeding initiation has increased, so have readmissions for hyperbilirubinemia, leading physicians to blame breastfeeding, instead of *mismanaged* breastfeeding. We are also putting parents in a difficult position by asking for both breastfeeding and exclusive breastfeeding (Figure 3.1), knowing that breastfed infants tend to have higher bilirubin levels (Gartner & Herschel, 2001). We must remember that the optimally breastfed infant is the *normal* in regards to bilirubin levels, not the formula-fed infant (Figure 3.2).

The Parental Paradox

Breast is best.

  Artificial feeding is hazardous to health.

Breastfed babies are more likely to become severely jaundiced than formula-fed babies.

  Severe jaundice can lead to brain damage.

But we want you to breastfeed, and breastfeed exclusively.

Figure 3.1. The Parental Paradox

Bilirubin Levels in Breastfed, Artificially-Fed, and Asian Infants

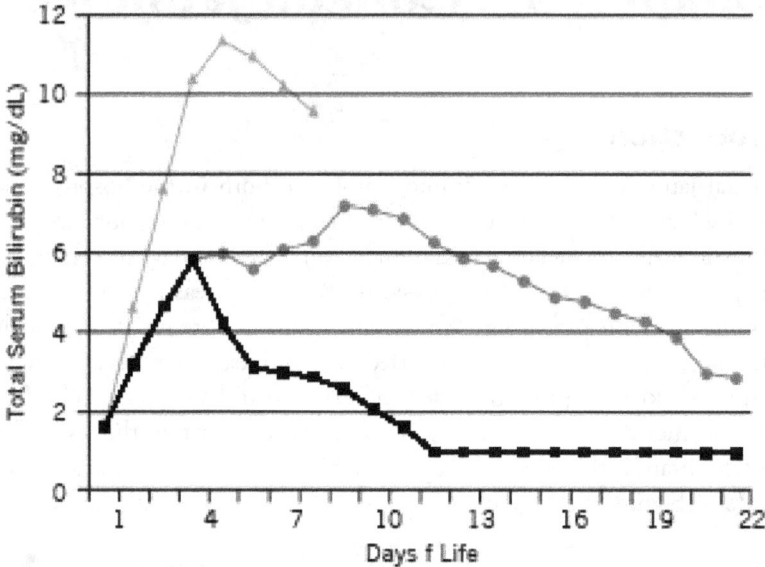

Three typical patterns of total serum bilirubin during neonatal jaundice in the earlt weeks of life are illustrated.

- ■ Full-term, healthy, artificially fed newborns
- ● Full-term, healthy, breastfed infants
- ▲ Full-term, healthy infants of Asian orgin

   *To convert bilirubin from mg/dL to umol/L, multiply the mg/dL by 17.1.

Figure 3.2. Bilirubin Levels in Breastfed, Artificially-Fed, and Asian Infants (Gartner & Herschel, 2001). Source: Gartner & Herschel, Pediatr Clin NA, 2001; 48(2):389-400. Used with permission from Elsevier.

Pediatricians in the U.S. often experience a "disease" called "Vigintiphobia," fear of the number twenty (20 mg/dL = 342 µmol/L)! Initial phototherapy and exchange transfusion recommendations to prevent brain damage were based on RH hemolytic disease research in the 1950s. The 20 mg/dL threshold for encephalopathy was shown NOT to apply to non-hemolytic jaundice in later studies. In the 1970's, phototherapy and exchange transfusions essentially eliminated reported kernicterus; however, there was considerable overtreatment and additional risks of exchange transfusions.

In the mid 1990's, a "kinder, gentler approach" was advocated by several authors (Newman & Maisels, 1992) and by the American Academy of Pediatrics (1994). Since this time we have seen an increase in readmissions for jaundice and a possible increase in kernicterus (permanent brain damage due to excess bilirubin), which have been associated with earlier discharges, lack of appropriate follow-up, and inadequate breastfeeding.

The MMWR (Centers for Disease Control, 2001) reported four cases of kernicterus from 1994 to 1998, with three of the four cases being "term," but 37 weeks gestation, and the fourth case an O/A incompatibility. The Joint Commission (JCAHO) also issued a Sentinel Event Alert in 2001 regarding an increase in reported kernicterus in healthy newborns (The Joint Commission, 2001). Also during this time period, there was an increase in late preterm infants (34 to 37 weeks gestation) (March of Dimes, 2011). Infants between 35 and 37 weeks have five to ten times the risk of readmission due to poor feeding, with resultant weight loss and jaundice (Edmonson, Stoddard, & Owens, 1997; Soskolne, Schumacher, Fyock, Young, & Schork, 1996).

A few definitions are in order. Jaundice is a yellow color to the skin or whites of the eyes. Hyperbilirubinemia is an elevated bilirubin for age. Acute manifestations of bilirubin toxicity (lethargy, irritability, hypotonia alternating with hypertonia, opistotonic posturing) in the first weeks after birth are termed acute bilirubin encephalopathy. The precise concentration of bilirubin and duration of exposure leading to neurotoxicity in any given baby is unknown. Most babies with severe hyperbilirubinemia escape without any apparent sequellae. Acidosis, dehydration, infection, and possible other unknown factors may be important in determining the development of acute bilirubin encephalopathy and kernicterus. Kernicterus is the chronic and permanent sequellae of bilirubin toxicity. Pathologically, it involves bilirubin staining of the thalamus and basal ganglia, with a severe form of cerebral palsy, auditory dysfunction, and intellectual handicaps.

Bilirubin Metabolism and Transport

Bilirubin is the catabolic product of heme-containing proteins, such as hemoglobin (most), myoglobin, and cytochromes. Bilirubin is synthesized in reticuloendothelial cells, released into the blood, and transported bound almost completely to serum albumin to the liver, where it is taken up by the liver via OATP (organic anion transporter) enzymes and conjugated to a mono- or diglucuronide via the UGT 1A1 enzyme (UDP-glucuronosyltransferase 1A1). Bilirubin glucuronide is excreted into the intestine, but is unstable and readily hydrolyzed to unconjugated bilirubin (Figure 3.3). The monoglucuronide is predominant in newborns and is more easily hydrolyzed to unconjugated bilirubin in the intestine. The unconjugated bilirubin is absorbed by the intestinal mucosa to return to the liver via the portal circulation. This process is called the "enterohepatic circulation."

Bilirubin Pathways

Bone marrow

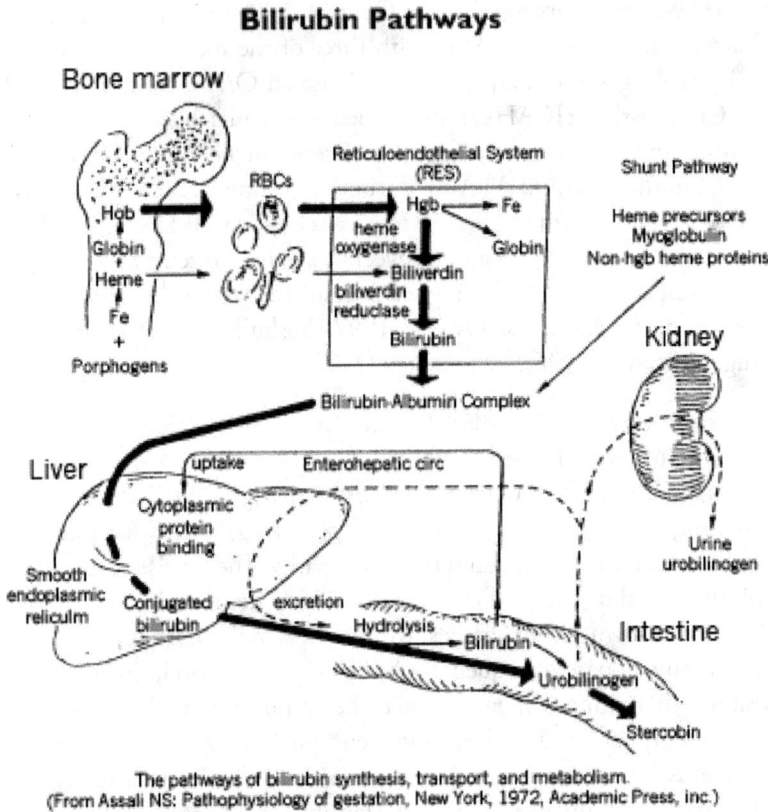

The pathways of bilirubin synthesis, transport, and metabolism.
(From Assali NS: Pathophysiology of gestation, New York, 1972, Academic Press, inc.)

Figure 3.3. Bilirubin Pathways. Source: Assali, N.S. (1972), Pathophysiology of gestation. New York: Academic Press, Inc.

There are several reasons why newborns have increased bilirubin relative to normal adult values ($\leq$ 1.5 mg/dL; 26 μmol/L). Higher values of unconjugated bilirubin result from a combination of increased bilirubin production from heme degradation, immature liver function, and increased intestinal reabsorption of bilirubin (Table 3.1; Gartner, Lee, Vaisman, Lane, & Zarafu, 1977). As bilirubin has multiple protective functions, the newborn normally has levels higher than children and adults. The antioxidant, anti-inflammatory, anti-apoptotic, and immune modulation properties of bilirubin have been associated with less peripheral vascular disease, less coronary artery disease, less cancer, less progression of amyotrophic lateral sclerosis, less severe atopic dermatitis, and better transplant outcomes in adults. The direct benefits to the newborn are less clear (Sedlak & Snyder, 2004).

Why so Much Bilirubin in Newborns?
Increased bilirubin synthesis in the newborn (compared with children and adults)
Shorter life span of red blood cells (RBC): 90 v. 120 days
Larger pool of RBC precursors in bone marrow, liver & spleen
Higher circulating RBC volume
Decreased liver function
Decreased hepatic uptake of bilirubin
Decreased conjugating capacity
Monglucuronide predominant form
Decreased hepatic excretion
Increased enterohepatic circulation
Increased hydrolysis of bilirubin glucuronide
Markedly increased concentration of β-glucuronidase in newborn intestine (10 X adult)
Meconium contains large amount of bilirubin
Influence of breastmilk (rich in β-glucuronidase)
Fasting physiology in the first few days of life

Table 3.1. Reasons for Increased Bilirubin in Newborns

Types of Jaundice

Physiologic Jaundice. In the first week of life, approximately 40% of healthy term infants will have total serum bilirubin concentrations greater than 5 mg/dL (86 µmol/L) and appear jaundiced (Bhutani, Johnson, & Sivieri, 1999). This normal elevation in unconjugated bilirubin is called "physiologic jaundice of the newborn." This physiologic jaundice must be differentiated from pathologic jaundice, which can be either conjugated or unconjugated and may be caused by infant pathologies, genetic factors, or drugs.

Pathologic Jaundice. Some populations have increased incidence and severity of jaundice. Both hepatic transporter and conjugation enzymes can have multiple mutations, leading to differing amounts and activity of the enzymes. Infants of Asian origin (including Native Americans) have higher peak bilirubins, peak slightly later, and retain jaundice longer (Huang et al., 2004; Saland, McNamara, & Cohen, 1974). Forty percent of Asian babies have a UGT mutation (G71R), and 10–20% of East Indian babies have a different UGT mutation (Huang et al., 2004). In Chinese newborns, one mutation increases the risk of severe hyperbilirubinemia 22 times, two mutations 88 times, with additional risk if the infant is breastfed. Gilbert's Disease is a specific mutation present in five to 10% of the U.S. population. It causes less UGT enzyme, which decreases the liver's ability to handle bilirubin, but it also provides some protection from coronary artery disease.

G6PD (glucose–6-phosphate dehydrogenase) deficiency is an X-linked enzyme deficiency (males primarily effected), with 500 known variations. It is present in 2–3% of Chinese, 4% of Greek, 13% of African-American, and 70% of Kurdish Jew ancestry, and offers protection against malaria. In the U.S., 21% of babies in the kernicterus registry had G6PD deficiency (Johnson, Bhutani, Karp, Sivieri, & Shapiro, 2009).

Pathologic jaundice is usually characterized by early appearance of clinical jaundice (before 24 hours of age), rapid rise in bilirubin (> 5 mg/dL per day), and total serum bilirubin greater than 15 mg/dL in formula-fed infants and greater than 17 mg/dL in breastfed term infants. Other factors include clinical jaundice persisting greater than two weeks and conjugated (direct) bilirubin exceeding 1.5 to 2 mg/dL, or greater than 10% of the total serum bilirubin (Table 3.2).

Causes of Pathologic Jaundice in Newborns

Unconjugated Hyperbilirubinemia:

Increased Production

Hemolysis

    Fetal-maternal blood group incompatibility

      Rh disease

      ABO incompatibility

      Minor group antibodies (c, Kell, etc.)

    Hereditary spherocytosis

    Other hemolytic anemias

      G6PD and medications

      Pyruvate kinase deficiency

      Thalassemias

      Other red blood cell enzyme deficiencies

Extravasation of blood

    Occult hemorrage

    Birth trauma

Polycythemia

Swallowed blood

Increased enterohepatic circulation

    Pyloric stenosis

    Ileus or bowel obstruction

    (Lack of breastfeeding jaundice)

Decreased Clearance

Inborn errors of metabolism

    Type 1 & 2 Gilbert disease

    Galactosemia

    Tyrosinosis

    Hypermethioninemia

Drugs and Hormones

    Hypothyroidism

    Hypopituitarism

    Lucey-Driscol syndrome

    (Breastmilk jaundice)

*Table continues on next page.

*Table continued from previous page.

Conjugated Hyperbilirubiemia:
Extrahepatic obstruction
Infantile obstructive cholangiopathy
Biliary atresia
Neonatal hepatitis
Choledochal cyst
Other causes
Extrinsic bile duct compression
Bile plug syndrome, etc.
Genetic and metabolic disorders (multiple)
Persistent intrahepatic cholestasis
Paucity of bile ducts, Byler disease, others
Acquired intrahepatic cholestasis
Infections
Drug-induced
Parenteral nutrition

Table 3.2. Causes of Pathologic Jaundice in Newborns

Breastmilk Jaundice. Breastfed infants frequently have unconjugated hyperbilirubinemia that extends into the second and third weeks of life, and often up to eight to 12 weeks of life (Alonso, Whitington, Whitington, Rivard, & Given, 1991; Gartner & Arias, 1966). In contrast to formula-fed infants, approximately half of all breastfed infants may appear mildly to moderately jaundiced past the first week of life. The prolongation of physiologic jaundice is known as "breastmilk jaundice" (Gartner & Arias, 1966). Research has demonstrated that two-thirds of transitional and mature human milk samples increase the intestinal absorption on unconjugated bilirubin in rats, presumably because of an unidentified substance in human milk (Gartner & Arias, 1966; Gartner, Lee, & Moscioni, 1983). Over time the jaundice and elevated bilirubin decline, but at a highly variable rate from infant to infant. Diagnosis of breastmilk jaundice is made in a healthy, thriving infant with good weight gain who exhibits jaundice after the fifth day of life. Other causes of jaundice must be ruled out. The treatment of breastmilk jaundice varies with the philosophy and judgement of the practitioner and will be addressed below.

Starvation Jaundice in the Newborn. Previously called "breastfeeding jaundice" or "lack of breastfeeding jaundice," this type of jaundice is actually the infant form of starvation jaundice. Lack of caloric intake in normal adults, even for only 24 hours, with good hydration, results in an increase in unconjugated hyperbilirubinemia of about 1–2 mg/dL (17–34 µmol/L) above normal adult values (1.5 mg/dL or 26 µmol/L; Whitmer & Gollan, 1983). In newborns, reduced caloric intake below the optimal for age, even without absolute starvation, results in greater increases in unconjugated bilirubin concentrations because of all of the developmental and physiologic factors listed on page 41 (Table 3.1; De Carvalho, Klaus, & Merkatz, 1982; Wu, Hodgman, Kirkpatrick, White, & Bryla, 1985; Yamauchi & Yamanouchi, 1990). Not all breastfed infants receive optimal milk intake during the first few days of life, which can result in increased bilirubin concentrations. The more frequently breastfeeding occurs per 24 hours, the less jaundice is seen (Figure 3.4).

Breastfeeding Frequency and Bilirubin

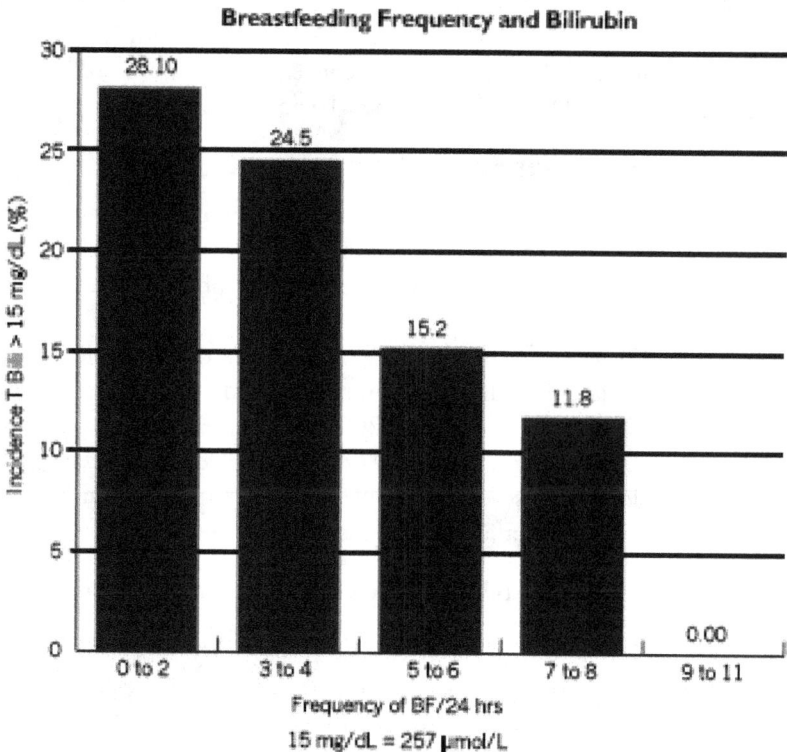

Figure 3.4. Breastfeeding Frequency and Bilirubin. Source: Adapted from Yamauchi & Yamamouchi, Pediatrics 1990; 86(2):171–175. Used with permission from AAP.

Two studies suggest that when breastfeeding is optimally managed, there are no differences in serum bilirubin concentrations in breastfed and formula-fed infants during the first five days of life (Bertini, Dani, Tronchin, & Rubaltelli, 2001; Dahms et al., 1973). However, the majority of reports indicate increased serum bilirubin and greater weight loss in breastfed infants (Maisels & Gifford, 1986; Schneider, 1986). Starvation jaundice is usually seen in the first five days of life and is NOT due to dehydration. Water supplements are ineffective at reducing bilirubin levels (de Carvalho, Hall, & Harvey, 1981). In this study there was no difference in the peak bilirubin levels in the no supplement group (15.3 mg/dL [262 µmol/L]) versus the water supplemented group (15.1 mg/dL [258 µmol/L]). There was a slight, but not statistically significant difference in the number of infants receiving phototherapy. The only parameter that was different statistically, but perhaps not clinically significant, was the mean weight loss of 6.6% in the no supplement versus 5.7% in the water supplemented group. Higher frequency of feedings (De Carvalho et al., 1982) and more frequent stools (Brodersen & Hermann, 1963) correlate with lower bilirubin levels in the first few days of life. Starvation jaundice and breastmilk jaundice can occur in the same infant, resulting in abnormally increased serum unconjugated bilirubin concentrations in the second and third weeks of life and beyond, which may be potentially toxic.

Breastfeeding-Friendly Management of Jaundice

Not all exaggerations of unconjugated hyperbilirubinemia in breastfed infants can be prevented, but close follow-up assures the detection and intervention for potentially toxic serum bilirubin concentrations (American Academy of Pediatrics, 2004; Gartner, 2010; Maisels & Newman, 1995). Breastfeeding is still perceived as a risk factor for severe hyperbilirubinemia, especially in late preterm and other high-risk infants (American Academy of Pediatrics, 2004). With early discharge and misguided breastfeeding management, poor feeding often goes unrecognized, leading to severe hyperbilirubinemia and well-meaning, but inappropriate supplementation or total discontinuation of breastfeeding.

Prevention of exaggerated bilirubin levels starts with optimal breastfeeding management. Following the Baby-Friendly Hospital Initiative 10 Steps (World Health Organization, 1989), the AAP Policy Statement on Breastfeeding (American Academy of Pediatrics Section on Breastfeeding, 2012), and the AAP Clinical Practice Guideline on Management of Hyperbilirubinemia, with the 2009 update (American Academy of Pediatrics, 2004; Maisels et al., 2009), breastfeeding is strongly recommended. These recommendations are summarized in the 2010 Academy of Breastfeeding Medicine Clinical Protocol # 22 and include early initiation of breastfeeding, exclusive breastfeeding (except when supplementation is deemed necessary —see Chapter 4), optimal breastfeeding management, education on early feeding cues, and identification of at-risk mothers and babies (Gartner, 2010).

Appropriate follow-up is essential. The AAP recommends every infant be screened at discharge with a transcutaneous or total serum bilirubin, which can be done at the time of the newborn screen. By plotting the bilirubin level on the Bhutani curve (Bhutani et al., 1999) by age in hours and by taking other risk factors into account, appropriate follow-up can be planned (Figure 3.5; Maisels et al., 2009).

Nomogram for Designation of Risk of Significant Hyperbilirubinemia

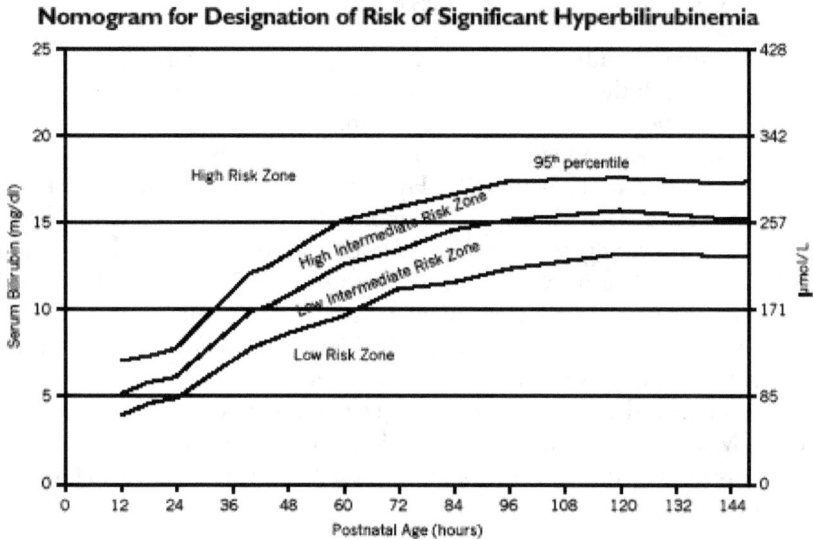

Nomogram for designation of risk in 2840 well newborns at 36 or more weeks' gestational age with birth weight of 2000 g or more or 35 or more weeks' gestational age and birth weight of 2500g or more based on the hour pecific serum bilirubin values. The serum bilirubin level was obtained before discharge, and the zone in which the value fell predicted the likelihood of a subsequent bilirubin level exceeding the 95th percentile (high-risk zone).

5 mg/dL = 86 μmol/L
10 mg/dL = 171 μmol/L
15 mg/dL = 257 μmol/L
20 mg/dL = 342 μmol/L

Figure 3.5. Nomogram for Designation of Risk of Significant Hyperbilirubinemia. Source: AAP Subcommittee on Hyperbilirubinemia, Pediatrics 2004; 114(1):297–316. Used with permission from AAP.

When efforts to prevent elevated serum bilirubin concentrations have failed, several treatment options are available: phototherapy, temporary supplementation with special formula, and temporary interruption of breastfeeding with replacement feeding with artificial baby milk. These management options may be combined and are compatible with continuing to breastfeed. Keeping mother and infant together as much as possible is a central goal.

Phototherapy can be done at home, in the mother's room, or in a special care nursery. Home phototherapy is possible, but discouraged, especially for infants with risk factors (American Academy of Pediatrics, 2004; Maisels et al., 2009). Breastfeeding infants readmitted from home for phototherapy should be admitted to a hospital unit in which the mother can also reside whenever possible, so breastfeeding can continue without interruption (Gartner, 2010). Interruption of phototherapy for up to 30 minutes to permit breastfeeding without eye patches does not alter the effectiveness of the treatment (Gartner, 2010). Recommended levels for initiating phototherapy are available in the AAP Guidelines (American Academy of Pediatrics, 2004; Maisels et al., 2009).

Supplementation of breastfeeding with cow's milk-based formulas has been shown to inhibit the intestinal absorption of bilirubin (Gartner et al., 1983). Supplementation of breastfeeding with small amounts of artificial infant milks can be used to lower serum bilirubin levels in breastfeeding infants (Wight, Cordes, & Chantry, 2008). Hydrolyzed protein formulas (elemental formulas) have been shown to be more effective than standard infant formulas in lowering serum bilirubin levels (Gourley, Kreamer, & Arend, 1992; Gourley, Kreamer, Cohnen, & Kosorok, 1999). Elemental formula does not expose the breastfed infant to whole cow's milk protein or soy protein, especially if there is a family history of allergies. In addition, elemental formulas taste terrible (the infant will want to go back to sweeter human milk) and are very expensive (the parents will not want to use it long term). Most importantly, supplementation with elemental formula conveys the message that this is a *temporary medical therapy*, not just switching to formula.

Why does artificial milk increase bilirubin excretion? Larger volumes of artificial milk are generally given in the first few days, leading to more rapid passage of meconium and less risk of starvation jaundice. The fat composition of formula may bind bilirubin and increase excretion. Lastly, elemental formulas contain an inhibitor of glucuronidase (L-Aspartic acid). However, is this more rapid than normal drop in bilirubin harmful to the infant?

Excessive amounts of formula should be avoided so as to maintain frequent breastfeeding and preserve maternal milk supply. If the mother is not producing adequate volumes of milk, the infant is incapable of transferring adequate milk, the infant weight loss is greater than 8–10%, or hydration is inadequate (based on both laboratory values and clinical signs), then larger amounts of formula should be offered to insure adequate caloric intake (American Academy of Pediatrics, 2004).

Temporary interruption of breastfeeding (24–48 hours) with full formula feeding will usually lower serum bilirubin concentrations more rapidly than supplementation, but may not be as effective as phototherapy (Martinez et al., 1993). With temporary interruption of breastfeeding, it is critical to maintain maternal milk production by teaching the mother to efficiently and effectively express her milk, so the infant returns to a good maternal milk supply. Mothers of jaundiced infants may be reluctant to continue or return to breastfeeding, and may need special support from healthcare providers to understand the importance of continuing breastfeeding.

Conclusions

Some degree of hyperbilirubinemia is normal and beneficial for all infants, with breastfed infants usually more jaundiced than formula-fed infants. Managing the intersection of jaundice and breastfeeding in a physiologic and supportive manner to ensure optimal health, growth, and development of the infant is the responsibility of all healthcare providers (Gartner, 2010). Current management of hyperbilirubinemia in a breastfeeding infant includes:

- Assessing the mother-infant dyad for risk factors for excessive hyperbilirubinemia.

- Assessing family history and ethnicity.

- Following bilirubin concentrations on an hour-specific nomogram.

- Determining the expected peak bilirubin.

- Following weights.

- Optimizing breastfeeding.

- Recognizing that parents will associate jaundice with breastfeeding and have increased anxiety regarding breastfeeding.

- Considering G6PD and other genetic causes of hyperbilirubinemia.

- Recognizing that late preterm infants (LPI) are at increased risk and consider a LPI protocol.

- Initiating phototherapy when indicated.

- Using expressed breastmilk, donor human milk, and artificial milk supplementation for appropriate indications.

- Insuring appropriate timing of follow-up.

Always remember, artificially-fed infants are generally *hypo*bilirubinemic when compared to optimally breastfed infants.

Chapter 4. Supplementation

Introduction

The goals of supplementation are to:

1. Provide the infant appropriate nutrition and hydration.

2. Avoid feeding-related infant morbidities (such as hypoglycemia, jaundice, and poor growth).

3. Establish and maintain a mother's milk supply, so the infant returns to breastfeeding.

Whereas other mammals provide adequate and nutritionally appropriate milk for their babies, we humans often feed our babies artificial substances made from another species' (cow's) milk. Given early opportunities to breastfeed, and breastfeeding assistance and instruction, the vast majority of human mothers and infants will successfully establish breastfeeding. Unfortunately, artificial milk supplementation of healthy newborn infants in the hospital is commonplace, despite widespread recommendations to the contrary (American Academy of Pediatrics Section on Breastfeeding, 2012; Wight et al., 2008; World Health Organization & UNICEF, 2003). Although any breastfeeding for a brief period has advantages over none at all, four to 12 months of breastfeeding is needed for many of the longer-term advantages to be realized. The most recent scientific evidence indicates that *exclusive* breastfeeding for the first six months is associated with the greatest protection against major health problems for both mothers and infants (Heinig, 2001; Kramer & Kakuma, 2004; Mihrshahi et al., 2007). In recognition of the importance of exclusive breastfeeding, the U.S. government has added *exclusive* breastfeeding targets to the Healthy People 2010 and 2020 goals (US Department of Health and Human Services, 2000, 2011).

Inappropriate Reasons for Supplementation in the Hospital

In the past (and still today) midwives, nurses, physicians, and other healthcare workers have suggested introducing water, glucose water, or formula to assuage thirst, maintain water homeostasis, decrease bilirubin, prevent hypoglycemia, "prepare" the gastrointestinal tract for digestion, calm a fussy baby, and relieve constipation, hiccups, or gas (Akuse & Obinya, 2002; Gagnon, Leduc, Waghorn, Yang, & Platt, 2005; Williams, 2006). Mothers with low confidence levels postnatally are very vulnerable to external influences, such as advice to offer breastfeeding infants supplementary or complementary foods–water, glucose water, or artificial baby milk (Blyth et al., 2002).

There are also many reasons why some women *choose* to formula feed or request supplementation in this early transitional period. The mother may feel she can get more rest if someone else can feed the baby. The mother may be ill. She may believe that she does not have enough breastmilk. She may feel she has to supplement immediately because she will be returning to work. Kurinij and Shiono (1991) surveyed reasons for in-hospital supplementation. The most common factors were associated with giving the mother more rest and convenience, but various permutations of "not enough breastmilk" came in second. "Hospital procedures" were also listed as a reason for supplementation for some patients.

A more recent study of in-hospital formula supplementation of breastfed infants from 150 low-income Washington, DC, families revealed that of the 60% who initiated breastfeeding, 78% received formula supplementation in the hospital (Tender et al., 2009). There was no clear medical need for supplementation in 87% of the infants receiving it. The reasons given for supplementation (Table 4.1) were similar to the earlier study. Infants of mothers who did not attend a prenatal breastfeeding class were almost five times more likely to receive in-hospital formula supplementation than those infants whose mothers had attended a class (OR 4.7; 95% CI, 1.05–21.14). An even more recent study (DaMota, Banuelos, Goldbronn, Vera-Beccera, & Heinig, 2012) addressed maternal requests for in-hospital supplementation of healthy breastfed infants of low-income women in California's Supplementary Nutrition Program for Women, Infants, and Children (WIC). Contrary to conventional belief, mothers' inaccurate expectations related to normal breastfeeding and infant behavior, rather than cultural factors, were the main reasons cited for supplementation in the hospital.

Maternal Reasons Given for In-Hospital Formula Supplementation	No. and Frequency (%)
Mother wanted infant to get formula	27 (39.1)
Mother unsure why infant got formula/ "nurses just gave it"	14 (20.3)
Mother felt she didn't have enough milk	12 (17.4)
Mother needed to rest	12 (17.4)
Infant illness	10 (14.5)
Doctor or nurse recommendation	9 (13)
Cesarean section and/or maternal medications	8 (11.6)
Poor latch-on	3 (4.3)

Table 4.1. Why Supplementation? Source: Tender et al, J Hum Lact 2009; 25(1):11-17. Used with permission from Sage Publications.

Unfortunately, there are many **inappropriate reasons** given for supplementation:

Colostrum is Insufficient. A basic lack of knowledge about, and distrust of, normal lactation physiology, often encouraged by formula literature ("breastfeeding is best, BUT, if you don't have enough...."), leads to the presumption that there is no milk or that colostrum is insufficient until the milk "comes in." As noted above, the small amounts of colostrum are normal, physiologic, and appropriate for the term healthy newborn as he/she learns to feed. Excessive supplementation often leads to emesis or "feeding intolerance" and a neonatal intensive care admission. In addition, in some cultures, colostrum is not understood or valued as a normal part of early breastfeeding and may be discarded in lieu of herbal teas or artificial milks until lactogenesis II (Morse, Jehle, & Gamble, 1990).

Prevents Weight Loss, Dehydration, and Hypoglycemia. The desire to prevent weight loss, dehydration, and hypoglycemia in the postpartum period is also part of this distrust of normal physiology. As we saw, there is a considerable body of research detailing normal weight loss in breastfed infants. A certain amount of weight loss is normal in the first week of life and is composed of both a diuresis of extracellular fluid received from the placenta and passage of meconium. There is now evidence that **too little** weight loss in the newborn period is associated with an increased risk of obesity later in life (Stettler et al., 2005). As discussed above, healthy full-term infants do not develop symptomatic hypoglycemia simply as a result of underfeeding (Williams, 1997).

Prevents Hyperbilirubinemia. This is a frequently cited reason for supplementation. An increase in bilirubin in the first few days of life is normal.

The more frequent the breastfeeding, the lower the bilirubin level (American Academy of Pediatrics, 2004; De Carvalho et al., 1982; Yamauchi & Yamanouchi, 1990). As bilirubin is a potent anti-oxidant (Kumar, Pant, Basu, Rao, & Khanna, 2007) and the appropriately breastfed infant has *normal* levels of bilirubin, artificially fed infants may be hypobilirubinemic!

Sleepy Baby. Being born is hard work for both Mom and baby! The sleepy baby who has had few feeds is a concern for both mothers and healthcare personnel. Here again, a trust in normal newborn physiology can lead to a decrease in inappropriate supplementation. Newborns are normally sleepy after an initial approximately two hour alert period after birth (Emde, Swedberg, & Suzuki, 1975; Stern, Parmalee, Akiyama, Schultz, & Wenner, 1969). Many times parents miss subtle feeding cues and expect crying as a sign of hunger. Also, maternal labor sedation or analgesia may interfere with breastfeeding. Trying to force feed a truly sleepy baby is usually frustrating for the feeder and the baby. Careful attention to an infant's early feeding cues and gently rousing the infant to attempt breastfeeding every two to three hours is more appropriate than automatic supplement after six, eight, 12, or even 24 hours. The general rule in the first week is "an awake baby is a hungry baby!"

Fussy Baby. The fussy or unsettled baby posses the opposite problem. Infants can be unsettled for many reasons. They may wish to "cluster feed" (several short feeds in a short period of time) or simply need additional skin-to-skin time (Wight, 2001). Filling (and usually *over*filling) the stomach with artificial milk may make the infant sleep longer (Matheny, Birch, & Picciano, 1990), missing important opportunities to breastfeed and demonstrating to the mother a short-term solution which will generate long-term problems.

Growth/Appetite Spurts. Growth spurts are periods when infants demand to nurse more (thereby stimulating an increased maternal milk supply), but excrete fewer stools, indicating more complete utilization of the available nutrition. These times are sometimes interpreted by mothers as insufficient milk. This may happen in later weeks, not in the immediate postpartum period in the hospital (Hillervik-Lindquist, Hofvander, & Sjolin, 1991).

Teach Bottle Feeding. Most mothers will have at least a few weeks at home with their baby before returning to work outside the home. Teaching a baby to take a bottle for later, while still in the immediate postpartum period is a specious argument. Because of the demand and supply physiology of breastfeeding, establishing exclusive breastfeeding is the first priority. After three to six weeks, when a full supply is established, bottles (or cups) of expressed breastmilk can be given by the father of the baby or others as needed.

Prevent Sore Nipples. In past years we have (in error) taught mothers to restrict the time at breast and gradually build up time to "prevent" sore nipples.

There is no evidence that limiting time at the breast prevents sore nipples. Sore nipples are a function of latch, positioning, and sometimes individual anatomic variation, like ankyloglossia, not length of time nursing. A study done 30 years ago (Slaven & Harvey, 1981) looked at timed and untimed suckling and found no difference in the incidence of sore nipples, cracked nipples, and engorged breasts, but a significant difference in mothers who were still breastfeeding at six weeks. The mothers who practiced timed feedings were breastfeeding significantly less (Table 4.2).

Unlimited Suckling Time Improves Breastfeeding at Six Weeks			
	Timed Suckling (n=100)	Untimed Suckling (n=100)	Significance P (C2)
Still breastfeeding	57	80	<0.0005
Hx sore nipples	33	38	NS
Hx cracked nipples	6	12	NS
Hx engorged breasts	37	27	NS

Table 4.2. Timed vs. Untimed Suckling. Source: Adapted from Slaven & Harver. (1981). Lancet, 317(8216), 392-393. Used with permission from Elsevier.

Maternal Rest. Letting the mother rest or sleep is a commonly cited reason for supplementation. We want the mother to rest while she is in the hospital because she is going to be extremely busy when she goes home. Well meaning healthcare professionals often offer supplementation as a means of protecting mothers from tiredness or distress, although this, at times, conflicts with their role in promoting breastfeeding (Cloherty, Alexander, & Holloway, 2004; Kurinij & Shiono, 1991). Helping mothers to breastfeed and explaining why a bottle may adversely affect subsequent breastfeeding often takes more time than actually giving a bottle or a cup (Cloherty et al., 2004; Smale, 1998). Also, healthcare professionals might find it difficult to justify time spent on relatively passive exercises, such as listening to and talking with mothers, as opposed to other more active exercises (such as bottle-feeding), which may be viewed more as "real work" (Cloherty et al., 2004; Smale, 1998).

Mothers are "programmed" to respond to their infants, and they get no more rest when the infant is away from them (Keefe, 1988). Keefe compared sleep quality and quantity in mothers whose babies were kept in the nursery versus mothers whose babies roomed in. The average hours of sleep were approximately the same. The mean quality of sleep was also comparable, with the mothers who were rooming in reporting slightly better quality and quantity of sleep. Interestingly, the number of sleep medications used was much higher when the baby was in the nursery!

It appears that nature programs mothers to wake periodically to check on their babies. There is no evidence that mothers will do better if baby is supplemented or away from the mother. Mothers lose the opportunity to learn their infant's normal behavior and early feeding cues if they are separated from their infants (International Lactation Consultant Assocation, 2005). It appears the highest risk time of day for an infant to receive a supplement is between 7:00 pm and 9:00 am (Gagnon et al., 2005).

Risks of Inappropriate Supplementation

What are the possible consequences of inappropriate supplementation? First, there is a significant impact on **gut flora**. Early supplementation permanently alters the pH of the gut to a more basic rather than acid level (Bullen, Tearle, & Stewart, 1977; Rubaltelli, Biadaioli, Pecile, & Nicoletti, 1998). Pathogens cannot survive well in the more acid breastfed gut, but thrive in the basic formula-fed/supplemented gut. We want to foster the growth of beneficial gut flora, not *E. coli* and *Pseudomonas*. There is also the potential for **sensitization to foreign proteins** and increasing the risk of developing allergies in susceptible infants (Host, 1991; Saarinen et al., 1999; Saarinen & Kajosaari, 1995; Vaarala et al., 1999). Inappropriate supplementation **increases the risk of diarrhea and other infections** (Chen & Rogan, 2004; Howie, Forsyth, Ogston, Clark, & Florey, 1990; Ip et al., 2007; Kramer et al., 2001; Paricio Talayero et al., 2006), especially where hygiene is poor (Edmond, Kirkwood, Amenga-Etego, Owusu-Agyei, & Hurt, 2007; Victora et al., 1987). In the Kramer trial (Kramer et al., 2001), the intervention hospitals were modeled on the Baby-Friendly Hospital Initiative 10 steps (World Health Organization, 1989), which includes no supplementation unless medically indicated (Table 4.3). The intervention hospitals' patients were much more likely to be exclusively breastfeeding.

PROBIT Trial			
	Intervention	Control	P or OR
Exclusive breastfeeding 3 months	43.3 %	6.4 %	p < 0.001
Exclusive breastfeeding 6 months	7.9 %	0.6 %	p = 0.01
Any breastfeeding 12 months	19.7 %	11.4 %	OR 0.47
Risk of GI infection	9.1 %	13.2 %	OR 0.50
Eczema	3.3 %	6.3 %	OR 0.54

Table 4.3. Supplementation and Breastfeeding Outcome. Data Source: Kramer et al. (2001). JAMA, 285(4): 413-420.

Supplementation in the first few days **interferes with the normal frequency of breastfeedings** (Kuhr & Paneth, 1982; World Health Organization, 1998), which can impact the establishment of a full milk supply. If the supplement is water or glucose water, the infant is at risk for **increased bilirubin** (de Carvalho et al., 1981; Kuhr & Paneth, 1982; Nicoll, Ginsburg, & Tripp, 1982; Nylander, Lindemann, Helsing, & Bendvold, 1991; Verronen, Visakorpi, Lammi, Saarikoski, & Tamminen, 1980), **excess weight loss** (Glover & Sandilands, 1990), **longer hospital stay** (Martens, Phillips, Cheang, & Rosolowich, 2000), or even water intoxication (Scariati et al., 1997). If the supplement is artificial milk, which is **slow to empty from the stomach** (Table 4.4; Cavell, 1981; Van Den Driessche et al., 1999) and often fed in larger amounts (Dollberg et al., 2001), the infant will breastfeed less frequently, as well (Matheny et al., 1990).

Gastric emptying in formula-fed and breast-fed infants			Half-emptying time (min)	
Author	Method	Age (Gest Age)	Breastfed	Formula Fed
Cavell, 1979	Marker-dilution	1-9 wk (33-38 wk)	25	51
Cavell, 1981	Marker-dilution	4 wk-6 mo (>37 wk)	48	78
Billeaud, 1990	Scintigraphy	0-12 mo (> wk)	61	76
Ewer, 1994	Ultrasound	0-4 wk (30-35 wk)	36	72
Van Den Driessche, 1999	^{13}C-octanoic acid breath test	1-10 wk (27-41 wk)	47	65

Table 4.4. Gastric Emptying in Formula-Fed and Breastfed Infants. Source: Van Den Driessche et al. (1999). JPGN, 29(1): 46-51. Used with permission from Wolters Kluwer Health.

The most significant risk of inappropriate supplementation is the **shortened duration of exclusive and any breastfeeding** (Blomquist, Jonsbo, Serenius, & Persson, 1994; Chezem, Friesen, Montgomery, Fortman, & Clark, 1998; Feinstein, Berkelhamer, Gruszka, Wong, & Carey, 1986; Hill, Humenick, Brennan, & Woolley, 1997; Howard et al., 2003; Kramer et al., 2001; Marques et al., 2001; Martens et al., 2000; Martin-Calama et al., 1997; Nylander et al., 1991). Studies have noted delayed lactogenesis II (also known as "secretory activation" or "milk coming in; Hartmann, Cregan, Ramsay, Simmer, & Kent, 2003) and maternal engorgement due to decreased frequency of breastfeeding in the immediate postpartum period (Moon & Humenick, 1989; Newman, 1990). Prelacteal feeds (as opposed to supplementation) are also associated with delayed initiation of breastfeeding and negatively associated with exclusivity and duration of breastfeeding (Perez-Escamilla, Segura-Millan, Canahuati, & Allen, 1996).

In one Swedish study (Nylander et al., 1991), the intervention group had early, frequent, and unsupplemented breastfeeding and the control group was given sucrose water and formula supplements. Duration of exclusive breastfeeding was examined at four time points. At three of the four points (1.5, three, and six months), there was a significant difference in the number of babies who were still breastfeeding, suggesting that supplementation does indeed affect breastfeeding (Figure 4.1).

Long term effects of a change in maternity ward feeding routines

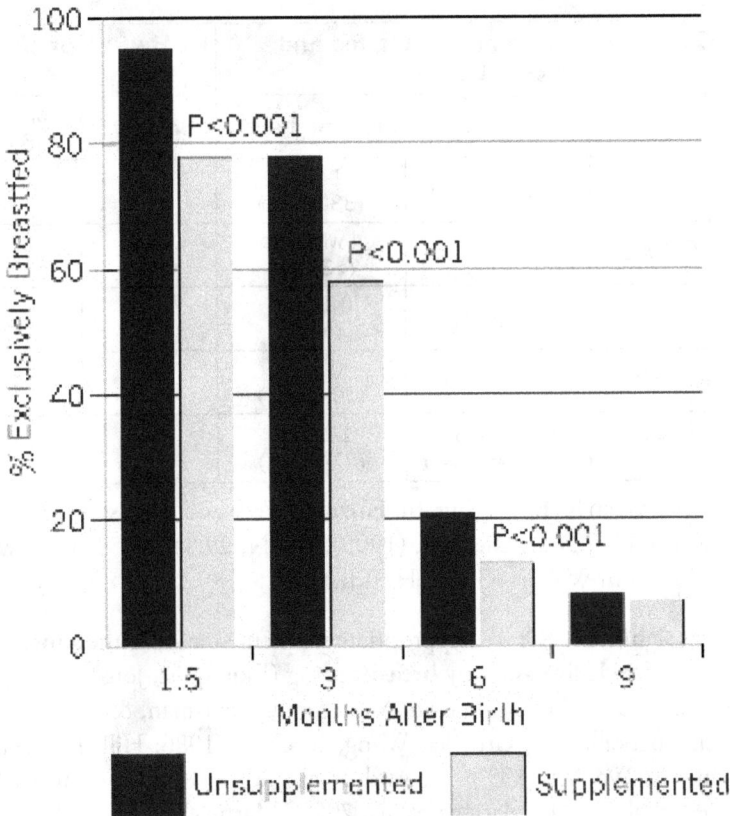

Figure 4.1. Outcome of Feeding Routines. Source: Nylander et al. (1991). Acta Obstert Gynecol Scand 70(3):205–209. Used with permission from John Wiley and Sons.

Martin-Calama et al. (1997) found that glucose water supplementation alone can also have an effect, not just formula (Figure 4.2).

Glucose Water Supplementation and Breastfeeding Duration

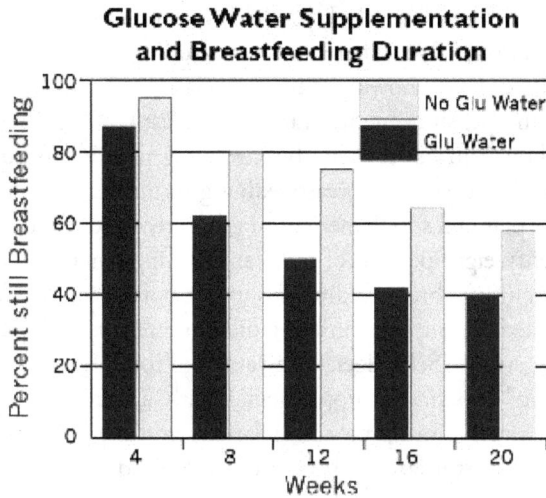

Figure 4.2. Glucose Water Supplementation and Breastfeeding Duration (Any Breastfeeding). Source: Martin-Calama et al. (1997). J Hum Lact, 13, 209–213. Used with permission from Sage Publications.

There are several other studies indicating early supplementation decreases duration of breastfeeding. Blomquist and colleagues (1994) studied 521 Scandinavian newborns: 69% of them exclusively breastfed and 31% supplemented with mom's own milk, donor milk (most), or formula (1%). Even in this very breastfeeding-supportive environment, 25% received supplementary feeds by day three. Indications for supplementation were: any birth weight less than 3 kg, maternal diabetes or gestational diabetes, insufficient amounts of milk, or infant fussiness. Supplementing in the hospital was high on the list of risk factors for not being breastfed at three months (Table 4.5).

Supplementary Feeding in the Maternity Ward Shortens the Duration of Breastfeeding	
Adjusted relative risk (estimated as odds ratios, OR) of **NOT** being breastfed at 3 months was associated with:	
Maternal age < 25 yrs	OR 4.2
Maternal smoking	OR 4.0
Supplements given	OR 3.9
Initial Wt loss ≥10%	OR 2.8

Table 4.5. Supplementation and Breastfeeding Duration. Source: From data in Blomquist et al. (1994). Acta Paediatr, 83(11), 1122-6.

If one reviews the Baby-Friendly Hospital Initiative documentation (World Health Organization, 1998), there are many studies, some well done, some not so well done, showing an association between in-hospital supplementation and shortened duration of breastfeeding. There are three studies that show "no" effect. In the Cronenwett study (Cronenwett et al.,1992), even the "exclusive" breastfeeding group received two bottles per week, while the planned supplementation group received five to nine bottles per week. Seventy-eight percent of the planned supplementation group and 74% of the "exclusive" breastfeeding group got bottles in the hospital. The authors concluded that supplementation did not interfere with breastfeeding! The Schubiger study (Schubiger, Schwarz, & Tonz, 1997) compared a "UNICEF group" (restricted supplements) with a "standard care" group. There were ten times more protocol violations and other crossovers in the UNICEF group. Most infants in both groups received one or more dextrose water supplements, as well as formula. There were liberal criteria for "indicated" supplementation, such as crying after breastfeeding. Only 8.3% of the UNICEF group were exclusively breastfeeding. The authors concluded that bottles and pacifiers made no difference!

Gray-Donald et al. (Gray-Donald, Kramer, Munday, & Leduc, 1985) came to a very interesting conclusion. They had two groups: planned supplements at 2:00 am and an "exclusively breastfeeding" group. Both the "exclusively breastfeeding" and the planned supplemental formula by bottle group got unlimited water and glucose water in the hospital. The authors concluded formula supplementation did not affect breastfeeding! The control group (unrestricted supplementation) infants who were *unsupplemented* were far more likely to be breastfeeding at four to nine weeks. It appears that formula supplementation in the hospital may be a *marker*, rather than a cause of breastfeeding difficulty.

In a study of 1085 women with prenatal intentions to breastfeed for more than two months who initiated breastfeeding, specific Baby-Friendly (World Health Organization, 1989) practices were evaluated (DiGirolamo, Grummer-Strawn, & Fein, 2001). The strongest predictors of breastfeeding termination before six weeks were delayed initiation of breastfeeding and in-hospital supplementation (Figure 4.3).

Percent of women who stopped breastfeeding
before 6 weeks, by specific hospital practices

■ Practice NOT Present   □ Practice Present

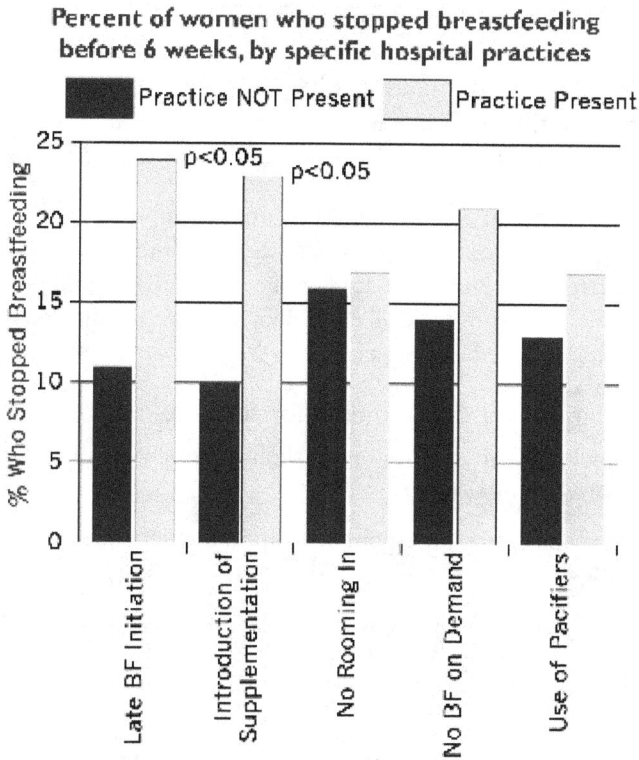

Figure 4.3. Stopping Breastfeeding by Hospital Practices. Source: DiGirolamo et al, (CDC). (2001). Birth, 28(2);94–100. Used with permission from John Wiley and Sons.

Inappropriate in-hospital supplementation is a predictor of shortened exclusive and any breastfeeding in many studies and appears to be one of the *most* powerful of the Baby-Friendly Hospital Initiative (BFHI) Ten Steps (WHO/UNICEF, 1989). In one of the papers from the Belarus study above (Kramer et al., 2001), the BFHI intervention group was more likely to be exclusively breastfeeding at three and six months. Studies in Brazil, Switzerland, Sweden, Scotland and further study in the U.S., confirm higher duration and duration rates when the BFHI steps are in place in the hospital (Braun et al., 2003; Broadfoot, Britten, Tappin, & MacKenzie, 2005; Hofvander, 2005; Merten, Dratva, & Ackermann-Liebrich, 2005; Phillipp et al., 2001).

Valid Medical Indications for Supplementation

There are a few valid reasons for supplementation. Powers & Slusser (Powers, 1999; Powers & Slusser, 1997) and the World Health Organization (1992) provide comprehensive lists of both maternal and infant indications for supplementation. The World Health Organization (WHO) updated its annex to the Global Criteria for the Baby-Friendly Hospital Initiative: "Acceptable Medical Reasons for Supplementation" (World Health Organization, 1992). The annex has been broadened to acceptable reasons for use of breastmilk substitutes in all infants. The handout (# 4.5) is the last few pages and available at: http://www.who.int/nutrition/topics/BFHI.

With every reason for supplementation, it is assumed there has been a complete evaluation of the mother/infant dyad, including an observation of a breastfeeding. It is important to evaluate the mother's milk supply, the baby's latch, and the baby's overall condition. The breastfeeding process must be evaluated before further steps are taken (Wight et al., 2008).

Infant indications for supplementation include:

- Infant with an inborn error of metabolism preventing the use of lactose (e.g., galactosemia).

- True hypoglycemia, unresponsive to appropriate frequent breastfeeding (Wight, 2006; Wight et al., 2006).

- Significant dehydration (Neifert, 2001; Yaseen, Salem, & Darwich, 2004). This is unlikely to occur in the hospital, especially since babies are going home in 24 to 72 hours.

- A weight loss of 8–10% accompanied by delay of lactogenesis (day five or later). We saw earlier that the average weight loss was 6% and occurred on day three, not later. If a mother's milk is not increasing normally and the baby has already lost much more than 6%, this is an indication for supplementation.

- Delayed bowel movements. If the baby is still passing meconium stools by day five, his intake is inadequate. The baby needs more food (International Lactation Consultant Association, 2005; Neifert, 2001).

- Insufficient intake despite mother's adequate milk supply. This may be a baby who has a dyscoordinated suck, a neurologic problem, poor muscle tone, or a congenital malformation precluding direct breastfeeding. The late preterm infant often falls into this category.

- Hyperbilirubinemia related to poor intake or extreme hyperbilirubinemia (>20 mg/dL or >342 μmol/L) in a baby who is a thriving infant with breastmilk jaundice. This usually occurs after hospital discharge, not in the hospital.

- Premature babies and low birth weight (< 2500g) babies when sufficient milk is not available or nutrient supplementation is indicated.

Maternal indications for supplementation include:

- Delayed lactogenesis II (secretory activation) and signs of infant problems because mother's milk supply has not increased, especially by day five. Delayed lactogenesis and an inconsolably hungry baby.

- Intolerable pain during feeding unrelieved by interventions. A breast pump or hand expression may actually be gentler than the baby, especially if you have a very hungry or very vigorous baby.

- Unavailability of the mother due to death, severe illness, or geographic separation.

- Some maternal medications (Hale, 2010). There are very few medications that are contraindicated for breastfeeding mothers. Magnesium sulfate is *not* one of them. Metronidazole (Flagyl) is *not* one of them.

- Primary glandular insufficiency (primary lactation failure), as evidenced by poor breast growth during pregnancy and minimal indications of lactogenesis, breast pathology, or prior breast surgery resulting in poor milk production.

- Retained placental fragments are a rare cause of milk insufficiency. If the rapid fall in progesterone does not occur from complete delivery of the placenta, the full milk supply will not develop.

- Sheehan's syndrome. Women who experience a severe blood loss during the intrapartum period may have temporary pituitary insufficiency with resultant limited milk supply.

What to Supplement

Expressed human milk is the first choice for supplemental feeding (American Academy of Pediatrics Section on Breastfeeding, 2012; Wight et al., 2008; World Health Organization & UNICEF, 2003), but expressing sufficient colostrum in the first few days may be difficult. The mother may need reassurance and education if such difficulties occur. Hand expression may elicit larger volumes than a pump in the first few days and may increase overall milk supply (Morton et al., 2009). Breast massage along with pumping may also increase available milk (Morton et al., 2009). If the volume of mother's own colostrum does not meet her infant's feeding requirements, pasteurized donor human milk is preferable to other supplements (World Health Organization & UNICEF, 2003).

The physician must weigh the potential risks and benefits of other supplemental fluids, such as standard formulas, soy formulas, or protein hydrolysate formula, with consideration given to available resources, the family's history for risk factors such as atopy, the infant's age, the amounts needed, and the potential impact on the establishment of breastfeeding. Protein hydrolysate formulas may be preferable to standard artificial milks, as they do not expose the infant to whole cow's milk proteins, reduce bilirubin more rapidly (Gourley et al., 1999), and convey the psychological message that the supplement is a *temporary* therapy, not a permanent change to artificial feeding. They also taste terrible, so infants prefer the breast, and they are expensive, so parents are less likely to continue them at home.

Glucose water is rarely indicated, except as an "extender" for colostrum. D10W provides only six calories per ounce and gives the infant a sense of fullness without adequate nutrition. Formula provides protein, fat, and more calories for a more sustained increase in blood glucose and better nutrition, but exposes the infant to cow's milk proteins. Supplementing with glucose water is also associated with increased bilirubin levels, while formula, especially elemental formula, tends to decrease bilirubin levels. Glucose water does empty from the stomach faster, encouraging more frequent breastfeeding, while formula decreases infant interest in frequent nursing due to longer dwell time in the stomach. Formula can modify gut flora, increasing the risk of infection, while glucose water is unlikely to do so (Table 4.6).

What to Supplement (in order of preference):
Expressed mom's breastmilk
Pasteurized donor breastmilk
Protein hydrolysate formulas
Regular infant formula
Soy formula
Water or glucose water

Table 4.6. Supplementation Options

How Much to Supplement

In past years infants were commonly NPO for eight to 24 hours before feedings were initiated. Currently, overfeeding (with subsequent emesis and NICU admission for "feeding intolerance") appears to be very common. Infants fed artificial milks ad libitum commonly have higher intakes than breastfed infants (Dollberg et al., 2001). **Given that breastfed infants are the normal, artificially fed infants are being overfed.**

A few studies give us an idea of intakes at the breast over time. In one study the mean yield of colostrum (using infant test-weighing) for the first 24 hours after birth was 37.1 g (range 7–122.5 g), with an average of 6 g intake per feed and six feedings in the first 24 hours (Saint, Smith, & Hartmann, 1984). A similar study also using test-weighing revealed a mean intake of 13 g/kg/24 hours (range 3–32 g/kg/24 hours) for the first 24 hours, increasing to a mean of 98 g/kg/24 hours (range 50–163 g/kg/24 hours) on day three (Casey, Neifert, Seacat, & Neville, 1986). Yet another study (Evans et al., 2003) noted breastmilk transfer of 6 mL/kg/24 hours for day one, 25 mL/

kg/24 hours for day two, 66 mL/kg/24 hours for day three, and 106 mL/kg/24 hours for day four in healthy vaginally-delivered infants allowed on demand breastfeeding. Interestingly, the intake of infants delivered by cesarean section was significantly less on days two to four (Evans et al., 2003). In a study where there was no rooming in and infants were fed every four hours, the average intake was 9.6 mL/kg/24 hours on day one and 13 ml/kg/24 hours on day two (Dollberg et al., 2001). In all studies, the range of intake is wide, but always less than current formula feedings.

As there is no definitive research available, the amount of supplement given should reflect the normal amounts of colostrum available, the size of the infant's stomach (which changes over time), and the age and size of the infant. Based on the limited research available, suggested supplementation for term healthy infants are in Table 4.7, although feeding should generally be by infant cue to satiation.

Suggested Feeding Volumes by Age for Term and Late Preterm Infants			
1st 24 hours	24-48 hours	48-72 hours	72-96 hours
2–10 mL/feed	5–15 mL/feed	15–30 mL/feed	30–60 mL/feed

Table 4.7. Suggested Feeding Volumes by Age for Term and Late Preterm Infants

How to Supplement

When supplementary feedings are needed, there are many methods from which to choose: a supplemental nursing device at the breast, cup feeding, spoon or dropper feeding, finger-feeding, syringe feeding, or bottle feeding (Wight, 2001). Depending on the method of supplementation (Neifert, Lawrence, & Seacat, 1995; Wight, 2001) or the number of occurrences of supplementation (Bunik et al., 2007; Feinstein et al., 1986; Howard et al., 2003), an infant may have difficulty returning to the breast. Radiologic and ultrasonographic studies show that there is a significant difference between the oral movements of bottle-feeding and breastfeeding babies (Geddes, Kent, Mitoulas, & Hartmann, 2008; Nowak, Smith, & Erenberg, 1995; Smith, Erenberg, & Nowak, 1988). Because there is this difference in the way babies feed, does that necessarily mean that babies cannot successfully go back and forth between feeding modalities?

The terms "nipple confusion" or "nipple preference" have been used to describe the reluctance of a baby given bottles to go back to the breast (Figure 4.4). It is not a new concept. Babies are smart – they would rather breathe than eat. They protect their airway and adjust to the milk flow, learning to prefer one feeding method and flow to another. The difficulty seen breastfeeding after bottle-feeding in some infants may be due to the very adaptability of the infant in learning a non-physiologic suck-swallow pattern.

Nipple Confusion/Preference Definition: "An infant's difficulty in achieving the correct oral configuration, latching technique, and suckling pattern necessary for successful breast-feeding after bottle feeding or other exposure to an artificial nipple" (Neifert, Lawrence & Seacat. (1995). J Pediatr 126: S125-129).

Figure 4.4. Nipple Confusion

There have been many different artificial feeding methods used throughout history (Baumslag & Michels, 1995). Breastfeeding is the normal way to feed infants. *All* other methods are "alternate" feeding methods, including bottle-feeding. Although cup feeding is the most common way of feeding in developing countries, many other techniques have been tried: tube feeding, "finger-feeding," spoon, syringe, and supplemental nursing systems. Bottles are the most common "alternate" feeding system in the developed world, but there is a correct and an incorrect way to bottle feed as well. The correct position is with the baby in a semi-upright position, with the baby and the feeder facing each other. If we give supplements, we want to give them by the route that is most likely to facilitate establishing or restoring breastfeeding. The problem is, we have very little information (even on bottle-feeding) as to how effective these methods are in reaching our final goal of establishing full breastfeeding.

What is wrong with just using a bottle? There are several concerns regarding the use of bottles and nipples with breastfed infants. Bottle use is associated with a shortened duration of exclusive and total duration of breastfeeding (World Health Organization, 1998). A report by the Office for National Statistics in London (Foster et al., 1997) studied babies given bottles in the hospital and babies exclusively breastfed. More babies given a bottle in the hospital than exclusively breastfed stopped breastfeeding within two weeks (34% vs. 11%). Was the bottle the cause or the marker of breastfeeding problems?

We also know that bottle feeding is different physiologically and affects the development of the oral cavity differently than breastfeeding (Palmer, 1998). Is it possible we have so many children with braces because we are using bottles rather than breasts? One study (Labbok & Hendershot, 1987) noted that increased durations of breastfeeding were associated with a decline in the proportion of children with malocclusion, even after controlling for known associated variables.

Even in the 1950's dentistry literature, it was thought that breastfeeding in the first six months of life might control a person's facial contours for the rest of his life (Pottenger & Krohn, 1950). Good facial development was felt to be an essential stone in the foundation of good health. There may also be an association of bottle-feeding with a smaller airway and obstructive sleep apnea (Palmer, 1998).

The main advantage in supplementing without a bottle is the nonverbal message to the parents that the alternative method is *temporary*. The bottle is often seen as the beginning of the end of breastfeeding. Davis (Davis, Sears, Miller, & Brodbeck, 1948), looking at the effects of cup and bottle-feeding said:

"It is a well recognized clinical observation that it is usually difficult to get a ... baby to nurse successfully if the infant has been started on bottle feedings, presumably because of the greater ease with which milk is usually obtained from a bottle."

The cup feeding technique used in this 1948 study was to pour the milk into the infant's mouth rather than have the baby sip or lap it out of the cup. Even when fed in this manner, the technique was found to be very effective, very safe, and it prevented what they were trying to prevent – bottle propping (Figure 4.5).

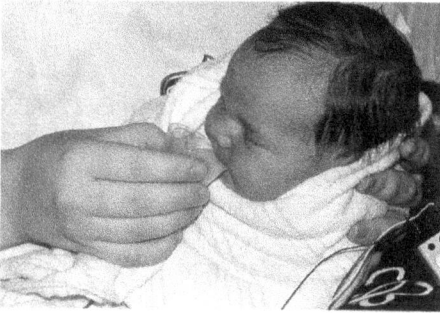

Figure 4.5. Cup Feeding

Cup feeding has been used throughout history. Current research confirms safety (Collins et al., 2004; Dowling, Meier, DiFiore, Blatz, & Martin, 2002; Flint, New, & Davies, 2007; Gupta, Khanna, & Chattree, 1999; Howard et al., 1999; Howard et al., 2003; Kramer et al., 2001; Lang, Lawrence, & Orme, 1994; Malhotra, Vishwambaran, Sundaram, & Narayanan, 1999; Marinelli, Burke, & Dodd, 2001; Rocha, Martinez, & Jorge, 2002; Schubiger et al., 1997), but we have little evidence that cup feeding is any more effective than a bottle or any other method in establishing full breastfeeding. In a randomized controlled trial of pacifiers and bottle or cup for supplementation, Howard et al. (2003) found that supplemental feedings, regardless of method (cup or bottle), had a large detrimental effect on breastfeeding duration. For those infants delivered by cesarean section, cup feeding significantly prolonged exclusive, full, and overall duration of breastfeeding. For those infants receiving less than two supplements, cup feeding prolonged exclusive and full breastfeeding; for those receiving more than three supplements, cup feeding prolonged exclusive, full, and overall duration of breastfeeding. As expected, those infants supplemented by bottle received significantly more total volume of supplementation (121 v. 67 mL) than cup-fed infants.

In a study of preterm infants starting oral feedings at a corrected age of 37 weeks in Brazil (rather late by U.S. standards), the authors found no significant differences between cup and bottle-fed groups with regard to time spent feeding, feeding problems, weight gain, or breastfeeding prevalence at discharge or at three month follow-up (Rocha et al., 2002). There was, however, a lower incidence of desaturation episodes in cup-fed infants. Another study of the mechanics of cup feeding in preterm infants (mean 30.6 weeks) found oxygen saturations stable, but in a 15 minute session, the average intake was only 5 mL, with 38% of the milk in the cup recovered on the bib (Dowling et al., 2002). Yet another study of preterm infants (Collins et al., 2004) found that cup feeding significantly increased the likelihood that a baby would be fully breastfed at discharge home, but had no effect on any breastfeeding at three and six months after discharge. It did, however, increase the length of hospital stay (cup 59 days v. bottle 48 days). Marinelli et al. (2001) found that cup feeding was as safe as bottle feeding for preterm infants, but takes longer and delivers less volume.

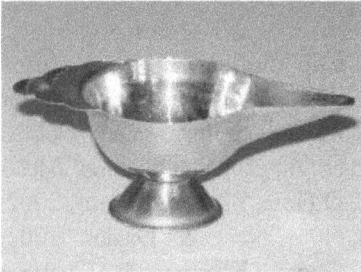

Figure 4.6. Paladi
Photo Courtesy of Chele Marmet.

Malhotra (Malhotra et al., 1999) studied 100 infants (66 term AGA, 20 term SGA, and 16 preterm) using the bottle, cup, and paladai (a small gravy boat shaped Indian feeding "cup"; Figure 4.6). Each infant served as his own control, as all three methods were given by the same caretaker. There was no effort to standardize the "technique" with any method (Table 4.8).

A controlled trial of alternative methods of oral feeding in neonates			
Parameter	Bottle	Cup	Paladai
ml/kg	11.6	13.1	14.0
ml/min	3.3	6.1	13.0
Spilling (%)	1.5	25.9	6.0
Satiety (hrs)	2.2	2.4	2.6
All differences statistically significant			

Table 4.8. Alternative Feeding Methods Trial. Source: Malhotra et al. Early Hum Dev 1999; 54:29-38. Used with permission from Elsevier.

The babies who had the paladai and the cup took slightly more than by bottle. The paladai appeared a faster method than either cup or bottle. The spilling was much worse with a cup. The paladai babies stayed asleep just a little bit longer. A more recent pilot study of paladai feeding (Aloysius & Hickson, 2007) demonstrated increased spillage, increased feed times, and more stress cues with preterm infants. Obviously, the exact technique with any method must be a factor.

Nurse midwives in Great Britain demonstrated that although the babies who were supplemented by cup were not statistically significantly more likely to be breastfeeding at discharge from midwife care, they were more likely to receive *any* breastmilk than the babies who were fed by bottle (Brown, Alexander, & Thomas, 1999). In another study looking at preterm infants and cup feeding (Gupta et al., 1999), 59 preterm and low birth weight infants were cup fed, with initiation of cup feeding occurring when swallowing was present (Table 4.9).

Cup-Feeding: An Alternative to Bottle Feeding in an NICU			
	28-30 wks on admit	31-34 wks on admit	35-37 wks on admit
# Cases	11	37	11
B Wt (gm)	900-1650	1350-2200	1750-2300
# Direct to Cup (%)	5 (45)	19 (51)	6 (54)
Age (days) at 1st cup feed (mean)	7-33 (12)	2-23 (7)	2-6 (3)
EGA at 1st cup feed (wks)	29-33.1	31.2-36	35.1-37
At Discharge: Direct BF only	3	22	8
At Discharge: Cup & BF	4	14	2
At Discharge: Cup only	4	1	1

Table 4.9. Cup Feeding in the NICU. Source: Gupta et al. (1999). J Trop Pediatr, 45(2):108-110. Used with permission from Oxford University Press.

The smallest and earliest baby in the study was 900 grams and 29 weeks. Of their total number of infants, 56% were discharged exclusively breastfeeding. Their conclusions were:

> *"Cup feeding is a skill that can be acquired by preterm infants at a stage when, developmentally, they are unable to breastfeed efficiently and when it is generally assumed that they require feeding by bottle."*

After reviewing the limited studies available, the Cochrane Database reviewers (Flint et al., 2007) concluded that cup feeding could not be recommended over bottle feeding as a supplement to breastfeeding because it confers no significant benefit in maintaining breastfeeding beyond hospital discharge and may increase hospital stay. There is little evidence about the safety or efficacy of most alternative feeding methods and their effect on breastfeeding; however, when cleanliness or refrigeration is suboptimal, cup feeding is the recommended choice (World Health Organization & UNICEF, 2003).

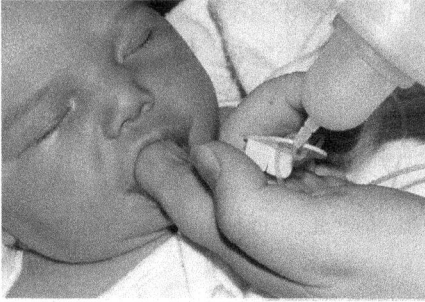

Figure 4.7. Finger-Feeding

There is even less information available about other methods of infant feeding. Oddy and Glenn (2003) studied finger feeding in the special care nursery in the context of a change to Baby-Friendly Hospital (BFHI) status (Figure 4.7). Breastfeeding rates at discharge increased from 44% before BFHI to 71% after BFHI implementation. However, finger feeding was only one of many changes.

Bottle feeding is the most commonly used method of supplementation in more affluent regions of the world, but is of concern because of distinct differences in tongue and jaw movements, differences in flow, and long-term developmental concerns (Wight, 2001). Some experts have recommended a nipple with a wide base and slow flow to try to mimic breastfeeding. Other researchers have tried to duplicate infant suckling mechanics (Geddes et al., 2008). At present the optimal feeding device has not presented itself and may vary from one infant to another.

When selecting an alternative feeding method, clinicians should consider several criteria: cost and availability, ease of use and cleaning, stress to the infant, whether an adequate volume of milk can be fed in 20–30 minutes, whether the use will be short- or long-term, the preference of the mother, and whether the method enhances the development of breastfeeding skills. No method is without potential risk or benefit (Cloherty, Alexander, Holloway, Galvin, & Inch, 2005; Wight, 2001). While one method may not be right for every baby, the "technique of the month" mentality should be avoided (Table 4.10).

Select a method to achieve specific therapeutic goals whether they are maximizing intake, retraining a poor suck, or supporting a mother's desire not to have bottles used with her infant. Feeding is not just nutrition. Convenience should not be **the** primary selection criteria. Cultural acceptability may be a major roadblock to some methods.

Advantages and Disadvantages of Various Supplementation Methods		
Method	**Advantages**	**Disadvantages**
Bottle	Familiar & socially acceptable Less time-consuming than most other methods Can measure amount Moderately inexpensive, widely available	Flow may be too fast Less infant control over feeding Associated with difficulties upon return to breast Long term use associated with orthodontic problems, dental caries
Cup	Inexpensive Easy to clean Baby or caretaker pacing Good eye contact, social stimulation Nothing but milk inside the mouth to cope with Encourages tongue protrusion and mouth movements Less fat lost than with gavage tube Stimulates olfactory and oral sensory receptors	Messy Imprecise as to intake Requires some skill and attention to infant cues Air swallowing requiring frequent burping Tendency to pour milk in Infant may develop preference for cup Infant doesn't associate feeding with the breast Does not fulfill infant's need to suck
Finger feeding	Can be used to correct disorganized suck Amount fed can be measured Baby or caretaker can pace feeding Anterior tongue position closer to breastfeeding	Harder to learn than cup More intrusive More equipment and increased cost Infant may become dependent on it May overwhelm babies with sensitive gag reflex Harder to clean Takes longer than cup
Dropper	No abnormal sucking Inexpensive Usually available Easy to learn Small amounts of milk placed anteriorly – low risk of choking	No sucking Difficult to clean Time-consuming Messy, imprecise Impractical for long term use

Advantages and Disadvantages of Various Supplementation Methods		
Method	**Advantages**	**Disadvantages**
Spoon	No abnormal sucking Easy to learn Inexpensive Easy to clean Small amounts of milk anteriorly – low risk of choking	No sucking Time consuming Hard to measure intake Impractical for long term use
Periodontal Syringe	Tapered tip with some sucking Can use with finger feeding or alone Can measure amount taken	More expensive Hard to find Hard to clean Time-consuming
Nursing Supplementer	Infant at breast, learning correct suck May encourage latch (immediate reward) Increased milk supply with nipple stimulation Allows measurement of supplement Baby-led pace of feeding Useful for infants with inadequate suck, tires easily, or needs extra calories	Awkward to use Moderately complex learning Hard to clean Expensive Hard to use in public Infant may learn to suck tube

Table 4.10. Comparison of Supplementation Methods

Supplemental nursing systems have the advantage of supplying appropriate supplement, while simultaneously stimulating the breast to produce more milk. Unfortunately most systems are awkward to use, difficult to clean, expensive, and require moderately complex learning (Wight, 2001). A simpler version, supplementing with a dropper or syringe while the infant is at breast, may be effective. For very short-term supplementation, the mother can hand express a few drops of colostrum into a spoon and feed it immediately. Cup feeding, finger feeding, supplemental nursing devices, droppers, spoons, and syringes are still unproven as to their effect on establishing successful breastfeeding long-term. However you choose, or a mother wishes, to supplement, the possible risks need to be explained to the mother and options offered her. It is not wise to force-feed babies who do not want to eat. There may be underlying pathology needing investigation if a full term, apparently healthy baby does not want to eat!

Supplementation Conclusions

If supplementation is needed, the indication, supplement used, and amount must be documented. When a mother requests supplementation or a bottle is given her infant, we should provide her with accurate information, and document the information given and the mother's response. The mother should be informed of potential risks and consequences. Many health professionals choose to use an information sheet; others use a consent form. A consent form may become a problem if the supplement is medically indicated, but the mother denies consent. Consult your facility attorney.

There are basic best practices that can minimize the need for supplementation. As a strong predictor of formula use is the delay in time between birth and initiation of the first breastfeed (Kurinij & Shiono, 1991; Smale, 1998), infants should be put skin-to-skin immediately to facilitate the first breastfeeding as soon as possible after birth (American Academy of Pediatrics Section on Breastfeeding, 2012; Saadeh & Akre, 1996; World Health Organization, 1998). Whenever possible, mother and infant should room-in 24 hours per day to enhance opportunities for breastfeeding and hence lactogenesis (American Academy of Pediatrics Section on Breastfeeding, 2012; International Lactation Consultant Association, 2005; Powers & Slusser, 1997; World Health Organization, 1998). Antenatal education and in-hospital support can significantly improve rates of exclusive breastfeeding (Su et al., 2007). And finally, all infants must be formally evaluated for position, latch, and milk transfer prior to the provision of supplemental feedings (American Academy of Pediatrics Section on Breastfeeding, 2012; International Lactation Consultant Association, 2005; Wight et al., 2008).

As we have seen, there are many reasons why infants are given supplements, most of them spurious. When supplementation is truly needed, it should be provided in a way to minimize the risk to future exclusive breastfeeding. The goals of supplementation are:

1. To provide appropriate nutrition and hydration.

2. To avoid feeding related morbidities.

3. To establish and maintain a mother's milk supply.

Anticipatory guidance regarding the normal course of breastmilk and breastfeeding should reduce the need for supplementation. With appropriate management of the early days of lactation, few infants should need supplementation.

Chapter 5. Hospital Policies & Procedures

Hospital policies and practices to support breastfeeding are critical for improving breastfeeding rates. Hospitals can either help or hinder mothers and babies as they begin to breastfeed. Hospital physical structure can affect breastfeeding rates by preventing the mother and infant from being together; although in most cases, there are possible solutions if the will is there. Much more important are the people who run and work in the hospital. They are the ones who determine hospital routines that either support (24 hour rooming-in, early feedings, on demand feeds, exclusive breastfeeding, no pacifiers or nipples, consistent and evidence-based advice) or discourage (maternal-infant separation, delayed and scheduled feedings, frequent supplementation, pacifiers, and anecdotal advice) breastfeeding.

As noted before, the Baby-Friendly Hospital Initiative (BFHI) 10 Steps have been associated with improved any and exclusive breastfeeding rates. The American Academy of Pediatrics (American Academy of Pediatrics Section on Breastfeeding, 2012), American College of Obstetricians-Gynecologists (2007), and American Academy of Family Physicians (2007) each have breastfeeding policies or statements supporting the BFHI recommendations. In 2007 the Centers for Disease Control and Prevention (CDC) began the mPINC census survey to characterize U.S. maternity practices related to breastfeeding (Perrine et al., 2011). The lowest prevalence of recommended practices were having a model breastfeeding policy (14.4%); limiting the use of formula, water, or glucose supplements for healthy full-term breastfed infants (21.5%; and providing adequate breastfeeding support to breastfeeding mothers at hospital discharge (26.8%; Figure 5.1).

Percentage of U.S. Hospitals with Recommended Policies and Practices to support breastfeeding, 2007 and 2009

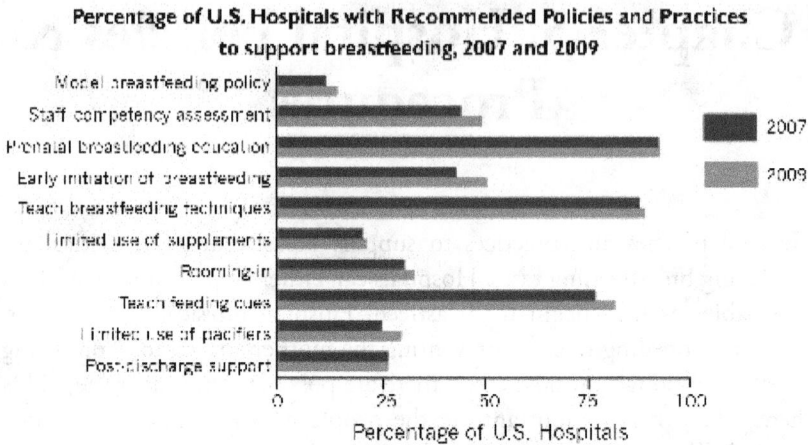

Figure 5.1. CDC–Percentage of U.S. Hospitals with Recommended Policies and Practices to Support Breastfeeding, 2007 and 2009. Source: CDC National Survey of Maternity Practices in Infant Nutrition and Care (mPINC) http://www.cdc.gov/vitalsigns/Breastfeeding/index.html

The CDC Vital Signs 2011 (Centers for Disease Control and Prevention, 2011) had several suggestions for hospital support of breastfeeding:

- Partner with BFHI-certified hospitals to learn how to improve maternity care.

- Use the CDC mPINC survey data to prioritize changes to improve maternity care practices.

- Stop distributing formula samples and marketing give-aways to mothers.

- Work with community organizations, doctors, and nurses to create networks that provide at-home or clinic-based breastfeeding support for every newborn.

- Become BFHI certified.

The CDC also recommended physicians and nurses:

- Help write breastfeeding-supportive hospital policies.

- Learn how to counsel mothers on breastfeeding during prenatal visits, in the hospital, and at physician office visits.

- Include lactation consultants and other breastfeeding experts on patient care teams.

- Coordinate lactation care between the hospital and outpatient clinic.

As most women make the decision to breastfeed before or during pregnancy (Noble et al., 2003), obstetric advocacy for breastfeeding can be very powerful

(DiGirolamo, Grummer-Strawn, & Fein, 2003; Lu, Lange, Slusser, Hamilton, & Halfon, 2001; Taveras et al., 2003). Obstetricians and family practice physicians can support breastfeeding by examining their patients' breasts and nipples, assessing for risk factors or past breastfeeding problems, and deferring hormonal contraception until breastfeeding is well established (around six weeks). Pediatricians and family practice physicians can encourage breastfeeding at prenatal visits, discuss the realities of new parenthood and breastfeeding, and provide support regarding other children and working outside the home. All healthcare providers can provide and recommend evidence-based appropriate education, correct misinformation, and encourage family and friend education and support.

Physician and nurse hospital practice can support breastfeeding by:

- Avoiding traumatic interventions (e.g., unnecessary suctioning).

- Placing the infant skin-to-skin with the mother.

- Allowing breastfeeding to take place (not forcing it).

- Delaying Vitamin K and eye prophylaxis until after the first breastfeeding.

- Managing visitors.

- Ensuring routine newborn orders are consistent with the BFHI Ten Steps (WHO/UNICEF, 1989) and AAP guidelines (American Academy of Pediatrics Section on Breastfeeding, 2012).

- Providing no discharge formula marketing bags.

- Providing lactation consultation as needed.

Hospital practice for neonatologists, pediatric critical care, or hospitalists should include:

- Prenatal neonatal consults that cover human milk and breastfeeding.

- Standing orders for lactation consult upon admission.

- Minimizing mother-infant separation whenever possible.

- Valuing any amount of milk.

Although a good start in the hospital is key, support for breastfeeding should continue after hospital discharge in the clinic or physician office. The high patient volume and limited time available for each visit in the outpatient setting presents significant challenges, some of which can be ameliorated by the use of lactation consultants. The American Academy of Pediatrics has developed many resources for the office setting and the American College of Obstetricians and Gynecologists has similar office tips.

Conclusions

For women who intend to breastfeed, the hospital experience is critical. To give infants the best start in achieving a healthy life, including reduced obesity, mothers must be supported immediately after birth. Suboptimal breastfeeding in the U.S. results in an estimated $2.2 billion in additional direct medical costs annually (Bartick & Reinhold, 2010). Recognizing the role of hospitals in helping women begin breastfeeding, Healthy People 2020 (US Department of Health and Human Services, 2011) added two objectives related to breastfeeding and maternity care:

- Reducing the proportion of breastfed newborns who receive formula supplementation within the first two days of life (MICH–23).

- Increasing the proportion of live births that occur in facilities that provide recommended care for lactating mothers and their babies (MICH–24).

Recognizing exclusive breastfeeding as a quality-of-care issue, the Joint Commission, the organization that accredits and certifies U.S. hospitals, added exclusive breastfeeding in the hospital as a new quality of care measure in 2010 (Joint Commission, 2011).

Hospitals provide care to nearly all women giving birth in the U.S. However, in most hospitals, this care falls short of evidence-based best practices that fully support mothers to be able to breastfeed. Supporting mothers through hospital breastfeeding challenges can help mothers reach their breastfeeding goals.

References

AAP, & ACOG. (2008). *Guidelines for perinatal care* (6th ed.). Elk Grove Village: AAP.

Adamkin, D.H. (2011). Postnatal glucose homeostasis in late-preterm and term infants. *Pediatrics, 127*(3), 575–579. doi: peds.2010–3851 [pii] 10.1542/peds.2010–3851 [doi].

Akuse, R., & Obinya, E. (2002). Why healthcare workers give prelacteal feeds. *European Journal of Clinical Nutrition, 56*, 729–734.

Alkalay, A.L., Klein, A.H., Nagel, R.A., & Sola, A. (2001). Neonatal nonpersistent hypoglycemia. *Neonatal Intensive Care, 14*, 25–34.

Alkalay, A.L., Sarnat, H.B., Flores-Sarnat, L., Elashoff, J.D., Farber, S.J., & Simmons, C.F. (2006). Population meta-analysis of low plasma glucose thresholds in full-term normal newborns. *American Journal of Perinatology, 23*(2), 115–119.

Alonso, E.M., Whitington, P.F., Whitington, S.H., Rivard, W.A., & Given, G. (1991). Enterohepatic circulation of nonconjugated bilirubin in rats fed with human milk. *Journal of Pediatrics, 118*(3), 425–430.

Aloysius, A., & Hickson, M. (2007). Evaluation of paladai cup feeding in breast-fed preterm infants compared with bottle feeding. *Early Human Development, 83*(9), 619–621.

American Academy of Family Physicians. (2007). *Breastfeeding, family physicians supporting (position paper)*. Retrieved from http://www.aafp.org/online/en/home/policy/policies/b/breastfeedingpositionpaper.html.

American Academy of Pediatrics Provisional Committee for Quality Improvement and Subcommittee on Hyperbilirubinemia. (1994). Practice parameter: Management of hyperbilirubinemia in the health term newborn. *Pediatrics, 94*(4), 558–565.

American Academy of Pediatrics. (2004). Management of hyperbilirubinemia in the newborn infant 35 or more weeks of gestation. *Pediatrics, 114*(1), 297–316.

American Academy of Pediatrics Committee on Fetus and Newborn. (1993). Routine evaluation of blood pressure, hematocrit, and glucose in newborns. *Pediatrics, 92*, 474–476.

American Academy of Pediatrics Section On Breastfeeding. (2012). Policy statement: Breastfeeding and the use of human milk. *Pediatrics, 129*(3), e827–841. Available from http://pediatrics.aappublications.org/content/129/3/e827.full.pdf+html.

American College of Obstetrician-Gynecologists. (2007). Breastfeeding: Maternal and infant aspects, Educational Bulletin # 361, February. Retrieved from http://www.acog.org/~/media/Departments/Health%20Care%20for%20 Underserved%20Women/clinicalReviewv12i1s.pdf?dmc=1&ts=2012052 3T0037432400.

Baby-Friendly USA. (2011). *The ten steps to successful breastfeeding*. Retrieved August 27, 2011, from http://www.babyfriendlyusa.org/eng/10steps.html.

Bartick M, & Reinhold A. (2010). The burden of suboptimal breastfeeding in the United States: a pediatric cost analysis. *Pediatrics, 125*, e1048–1056.

Baumslag, N., & Michels, D. (1995). *Milk, money, and madness*. Westport, CT: Bergin & Garvey.

Bertini, G., Dani, C., Tronchin, M., & Rubaltelli, F.F. (2001). Is breastfeeding really favoring early neonatal jaundice? *Pediatrics, 107*(3), E41.

Bhutani, V.K., Johnson, L., & Sivieri, E.M. (1999). Predictive ability of a predischarge hour-specific serum bilirubin for subsequent significant hyperbilirubinemia in healthy term and near-term newborns. *Pediatrics, 103*(1), 6–14.

Blomquist, H.K., Jonsbo, F., Serenius, F., & Persson, L.A. (1994). Supplementary feeding in the maternity ward shortens the duration of breast feeding. *Acta Paediatrica, 83*(11), 1122–1126.

Blyth, R., Creedy, D., Dennis, C., Moyle, W., Pratt, J., & DeVries, S. (2002). Effect of maternal confidence on breastfeeding duration: An application of breastfeeding self-efficacy theory. *Birth, 29*(4), 278–284.

Boluyt, N., van Kempen, A., & Offringa, M. (2006). Neurodevelopment after neonatal hypoglycemia: A systematic review and design of an optimal future study. *Pediatrics, 117*(6), 2231–2243. doi: 117/6/2231 [pii] 10.1542/ peds.2005-1919 [doi].

Brand, P.L., Molenaar, N.L., Kaaijk, C., & Wierenga, W.S. (2005). Neurodevelopmental outcome of hypoglycaemia in healthy, large for gestational age, term newborns. *Archives of Disease in Childhood, 90*(1), 78–81. doi: 90/1/78 [pii] 10.1136/adc.2003.039412 [doi].

Braun, M. L., Giugliani, E. R., Soares, M. E., Giugliani, C., de Oliveira, A. P., & Danelon, C. M. (2003). Evaluation of the impact of the baby-friendly hospital initiative on rates of breastfeeding. *American Journal of Public Health, 93*(8), 1277–1279. doi: 10.2105/AJPH.93.8.1277.

Broadfoot, M., Britten, J., Tappin, D. M., & MacKenzie, J. M. (2005). The Baby Friendly Hospital Initiative and breast feeding rates in Scotland. *Archives of Disease in Childhood. Fetal and Neonatal Edition, 90*(2), F114–116. doi: 90/2/ F114 [pii] 10.1136/adc.2003.041558.

Brodersen, R., & Hermann, L. S. (1963). Intestinal reabsorption of unconjugated bilirubin. A possible contributing factor in neonatal jaundice. *Lancet, 1*(7293), 1242.

Brown, S.J., Alexander, J., & Thomas, P. (1999). Feeding outcome in breast-fed term babies supplemented by cup or bottle. *Midwifery, 15*(2), 92–96.

Bullen, C., Tearle, P., & Stewart, M. (1977). The effect of "humanized" milks and supplemented breast feeding on the faecal flora of infants. *Journal of Medical Microbiology, 10*(4), 403–413.

Bunik, M., Beaty, B., Dickinson, M., Shobe, P., Kempe, A., & O'Connor, M. (2007, Oct 12–14). *Early formula supplementation in breastfeeding mothers: How much is too much for breastfeeding success? Abstract # 18.* Paper presented at the 12th Annual International Meeting of the Academy of Breastfeeding Medicine: Frontiers in Breastfeeding Medicine, Ft. Worth, Texas.

California Breastfeeding Promotion Advisory Committee. (2007). Breastfeeding: Investing in California's future. Breastfeeding Promotion Advisory Committee Report to the California Department of Health Services, Primary Care, and Family Health Division. Retrieved from http://www.cdph.ca.gov/ programs/breastfeeding/Pages/BreastfeedingInvestinginCalifornia Future.aspx.

Casey, C.E., Neifert, M.R., Seacat, J.M., & Neville, M.C. (1986). Nutrient intake by breast-fed infants during the first five days after birth. *American Journal of Diseases of Children, 140*(9), 933–936.

Cavell, B. (1981). Gastric emptying in infants fed human milk or infant formula. *Acta Paediatrica Scandinavica, 70*, 639–641.

Centers for Disease Control and Prevention. (2011). Hospital support for breastfeeding. *CDC Vital Signs,* (August 2011). Retrieved from http://www. cdc.gov/vitalsigns/Breastfeeding/index.html.

Centers for Disease Control (2001). Kernicterus in full-term infants—United States, 1994–1998. *MMWR Morbity & Mortality Weekly Report, 50*(23), 491–494.

Chantry, C.J., Nommsen-Rivers, L.A., Peerson, J.M., Cohen, R.J., & Dewey, K.G. (2011). Excess weight loss in first-born breastfed newborns relates to maternal intrapartum fluid balance. *Pediatrics, 127*(1), e171–179. doi: peds.2009-2663 [pii] 10.1542/peds.2009-2663 [doi].

Chen, A., & Rogan, W.J. (2004). Breastfeeding and the risk of postneonatal death in the United States. *Pediatrics, 113*(5), e435–439.

Chezem, J., Friesen, C., Montgomery, P., Fortman, T., & Clark, H. (1998). Lactation duration: Influences of human milk replacements and formula samples on women planning postpartum employment. *Journal of Obstetric, Gynecologic, and Neonatal Nursing, 27*(6), 646–651.

Cloherty, M., Alexander, J., & Holloway, I. (2004). Supplementing breast-fed babies in the UK to protect their mothers from tiredness or distress. *Midwifery, 20*(2), 194–204.

Cloherty, M., Alexander, J., Holloway, I., Galvin, K., & Inch, S. (2005). The cup-versus-bottle debate: A theme from an ethnographic study of the supplementation of breastfed infants in hospital in the United kingdom. *Journal of Human Lactation, 21*(2), 151–162; quiz 163–156.

Cohen, R.J., Brown, K., Rivera, L., & Dewey, K. (2000). Exclusively breastfed, low birth weight term infants do not need supplemental water. *Acta Paediatrica, 89*, 550–552.

Cole, M.D., & Peevy, K. (1994). Hypoglycemia in normal neonates appropriate for gestational age. *Journal of Perinatology, 14*(2), 118–120.

Collins, C.T., Ryan, P., Crowther, C.A., McPhee, A.J., Paterson, S., & Hiller, J.E. (2004). Effect of bottles, cups, and dummies on breast feeding in preterm infants: a randomised controlled trial. *BMJ, 329*(7459), 193–198.

Cornblath M., & Schwartz R. (1991). *Disorders of carbohydrate metabolism in infancy* (3rd ed.). Boston: Blackwell Scientific.

Cornblath, M., Hawdon, J.M., Williams, A.F., Aynsley-Green, A., Ward-Platt, M.P., Schwartz, R., & Kalhan, S.C. (2000). Controversies regarding definition of neonatal hypoglycemia: Suggested operational thresholds. *Pediatrics, 105*(5), 1141–1145.

Cornblath, M., & Ichord, R. (2000). Hypoglycemia in the neonate. *Seminars in Perinatology, 24*(2), 136–149.

Cornblath, M., & Reisner, S.H. (1965). Blood glucose in the neonate and its clinical significance. *New England Journal of Medicine, 273*(7), 378–381.

Cowett, R.M., & Loughead, J.L. (2002). Neonatal glucose metabolism: Differential diagnoses, evaluation, and treatment of hypoglycemia. *Neonatal Network, 21*(4), 9–19.

Cronenwett, L., Stukel, T., Kearney, M., Barrett, J., Covington, C., Del Monte, K., ... Rippe, L. (1992). Single daily bottle use in the early weeks postpartum and breast-feeding outcomes. *Pediatrics, 90*(5), 760–766.

Crossland, D.S., Richmond, S., Hudson, M., Smith, K., & Abu-Harb, M. (2008). Weight change in the term baby in the first 2 weeks of life. *Acta Paediatrica, 97*(4), 425–429. doi: APA685 [pii] 10.1111/j.1651-2227. 2008.00685.x [doi].

Dahlberg, M., & Whitelaw, A. (1997). Evaluation of HemoCue Blood Glucose Analyzer for the instant diagnosis of hypoglycaemia in newborns. *Scandinavian Journal of Clinical and Laboratory Investigation, 57*(8), 719–724.

Dahms, B.B., Krauss, A.N., Gartner, L.M., Klain, D.B., Soodalter, J., & Auld, P.A. (1973). Breast feeding and serum bilirubin values during the first 4 days of life. *Journal of Pediatrics, 83*(6), 1049–1054.

DaMota, K., Banuelos, J., Goldbronn, J., Vera-Beccera, L.E., & Heinig, M.J. (2012). Maternal request for in-hopsital supplementation of healthy breastfed infants among low-income women. J Hum Lact; published online 24 May 2012; doi: 10.1177/0890334412445299. Retrieved from http://jhl.sagepub.com/content/early/2012/05/23/0890334412445299.

Davanzo, R., Cannioto, Z., Ronfani, L., Monasta, L., & Demarini, S. Breastfeeding and neonatal weight loss in healthy term infants. J Hum Lact; published online 3 May 2012; doi 10.1177/0890334412444005. Retrieved from http://jhl.sagepub.com/content/early/2012/04/26/0890334412444005.

Davis, H.V., Sears, R.R., Miller, H.C., & Brodbeck, A.J. (1948). Effects of cup, bottle and breast feeding on oral activities of newborn infants. *Pediatrics, 2,* 549–558.

de Carvalho, M., Hall, M., & Harvey, D. (1981). Effects of water supplementation on physiological jaundice in breast-fed babies. *Archives of Diseases in Childhood, 56*(7), 568–569.

De Carvalho, M., Klaus, M.H., & Merkatz, R.B. (1982). Frequency of breast-feeding and serum bilirubin concentration. *American Journal of Diseases of Children, 136*(8), 737–738.

de Lonlay, P., Giurgea, I., Touati, G., & Saudubray, J.M. (2004). Neonatal hypoglycaemia: Aetiologies. *Seminars in Neonatology, 9*(1), 49–58. doi: 10.1016/j.siny.2003.08.002 [doi] S108427560300126X [pii].

DiGirolamo A, Thompson N, Martorell R, Fein S, & Grummer-Strawn L. (2005). Intention or Experience? Predictors of continued breastfeeding. *Health Education & Behavior, 32*, 208–226.

DiGirolamo, A.M., Grummer-Strawn, L.M., & Fein, S. (2001). Maternity care practices: Implications for breastfeeding. *Birth, 28*(2), 94–100.

DiGirolamo, A.M., Grummer-Strawn, L.M., & Fein, S.B. (2003). Do perceived attitudes of physicians and hospital staff affect breastfeeding decisions? *Birth, 30*(2), 94–100.

Dollberg, S., Lahav, S., & Mimouni, F.B. (2001). A comparison of intakes of breast-fed and bottle-fed infants during the first two days of life. *Journal of the American College of Nutrition, 20*(3), 209–211.

Dowling, D.A., Meier, P.P., DiFiore, J.M., Blatz, M., & Martin, R.J. (2002). Cup-feeding for preterm infants: Mechanics and safety. *Journal of Human Lactation, 18*(1), 13–20; quiz 46–19, 72.

Durand, R., Hodges, S., LaRock, S., Lund. L., Schmid, S., Swick, D., et al. (1997). The effect of skin-to-skin breast-feeding in the immediate recovery period on newborn thermoregulation and blood glucose values. *Neonatal Intensive Care, March- April*, 23–29.

Edmond, J., Auestad, N., Robbins, R.A., & Bergstrom, J.D. (1985). Ketone body metabolism in the neonate: Development and the effect of diet. *Federation Proceedings, 44*(7), 2359–2364.

Edmond, K.M., Kirkwood, B.R., Amenga-Etego, S., Owusu-Agyei, S., & Hurt, L.S. (2007). Effect of early infant feeding practices on infection-specific neonatal mortality: An investigation of the causal links with observational data from rural Ghana. *American Journal of Clinical Nutrition, 86*(4), 1126–1131.

Edmonson, M.B., Stoddard, J.J., & Owens, L.M. (1997). Hospital readmission with feeding-related problems after early postpartum discharge of normal newborns. *The Journal of the American Medical Association, 278*(4), 299–303.

Eidelman, A.I. (2001). Hypoglycemia and the breastfed neonate. *Pediatric Clinics of North America, 48*(2), 377–387.

Ellis, M., Manandhar, D. S., Manandhar, N., Land, J. M., Patel, N., & de, L. C. A. M. (1996). Comparison of two cotside methods for the detection of hypoglycaemia among neonates in Nepal. *Archives of Diseases in Childhood. Fetal and Neonatal Edition, 75*(2), F122–125.

Emde, R., Swedberg, J., & Suzuki, B. (1975). Human wakefulness and biological rhythms after birth. *Archives of General Psychiatry, 32*, 780–783.

Evans, K.C., Evans, R.G., Royal, R., Esterman, A.J., & James, S.L. (2003). Effect of caesarean section on breast milk transfer to the normal term newborn over the first week of life. *Archives of Diseases in Childhood. Fetal and Neonatal Edition, 88*(5), F380–382.

Feinstein, J.M., Berkelhamer, J.E., Gruszka, M.E., Wong, C.A., & Carey, A.E. (1986). Factors related to early termination of breast-feeding in an urban population. *Pediatrics, 78*(2), 210–215.

Feldman-Winter, L.B., Schanler, R.J., O'Connor, K.G., & Lawrence, R.A. (2008). Pediatricians and the promotion and support of breastfeeding. *Archives of Pediatrics & Adolescent Medicine, 162*, 1142–1149.

Flaherman, V.J., Bokser, S., & Newman, T.B. (2010). First-day newborn weight loss predicts in-hospital weight nadir for breastfeeding infants. *Breastfeeding Medicine, 5*(4), 165–168. doi: 10.1089/bfm.2009.0047 [doi].

Flint, A., New, K., & Davies, M.W. (2007). Cup feeding versus other forms of supplemental enteral feeding for newborn infants unable to fully breastfeed. *Cochrane Database of Systematic Reviews*, (2), CD005092.

Foster, K., Lader, D., Cheesbrough, et al. (1997). *Infant feeding 1995*. London, UK: Stationery Office, Office for National Statistics.

Freed, G.L., Clark, S.J., Sorenson, J., Lohr, J.A., Cefalo, R., & Curtis, P. (1995). National assessment of physicians' breast-feeding knowledge, attitudes, training and experience. *The Journal of the American Medical Association, 273*, 472–476.

Gagnon, A.J., Leduc, G., Waghorn, K., Yang, H., & Platt, R.W. (2005). In-hospital formula supplementation of healthy breastfeeding newborns. *Journal of Human Lactation, 21*(4), 397–405.

Gartner, L.M. (2010). ABM clinical protocol #22: Guidelines for management of jaundice in the breastfeeding infant equal to or greater than 35 weeks' gestation. *Breastfeeding Medicine, 5*(2), 87–93.

Gartner, L.M., & Arias, I.M. (1966). Studies of prolonged neonatal jaundice in the breast-fed infant. *Journal of Pediatrics, 68*(1), 54–66.

Gartner, L.M., & Herschel, M. (2001). Jaundice and breastfeeding. *Pediatric Clinics of North America, 48*(2), 389–399.

Gartner, L.M., Lee, K.S., & Moscioni, A.D. (1983). Effect of milk feeding on intestinal bilirubin absorption in the rat. *Journal of Pediatrics, 103*(3), 464–471.

Gartner, L.M., Lee, K.S., Vaisman, S., Lane, D., & Zarafu, I. (1977). Development of bilirubin transport and metabolism in the newborn rhesus monkey. *Journal of Pediatrics, 90*(4), 513–531.

Geddes, D.T., Kent, J.C., Mitoulas, L.R., & Hartmann, P.E. (2008). Tongue movements and intra-oral vacuum in breastfeeding infants. *Early Human Development, 84*(7), 471–477. *doi:10.1016/j.earlhumdev.2007.12.008.*

Glover, J., & Sandilands, M. (1990). Supplementation of breastfeeding infants and weight loss in hospital. *Journal of Human Lactation, 6*(4), 163–166.

Goldberg, N., & Adams, E. (1983). Supplementary water for breast-fed babies in a hot and dry climate–not really a necessity. *Archives of Diseases in Childhood, 58*, 73–74.

Gourley, G.R., Kreamer, B., & Arend, R. (1992). The effect of diet on feces and jaundice during the first 3 weeks of life. *Gastroenterology, 103*(2), 660–667. doi: S0016508592003512 [pii].

Gourley, G.R., Kreamer, B., Cohnen, M., & Kosorok, M.R. (1999). Neonatal jaundice and diet. *Archives of Pediatrics & Adolescent Medicine, 153*(2), 184–188.

Gray-Donald, K., Kramer, M.S., Munday, S., & Leduc, D.G. (1985). Effect of formula supplementation in the hospital on the duration of breast-feeding: a controlled clinical trial. *Pediatrics, 75*(3), 514–518.

Gupta, A., Khanna, K., & Chattree, S. (1999). Cup feeding: An alternative to bottle feeding in a neonatal intensive care unit. *Journal of Tropical Pediatrics, 45*(2), 108–110.

Hale T.W. (2010). *Medications and mothers' milk* (15th ed.). Amarillo, Texas: Hale Publishing.

Hamilton, B.E., Martin, J.A., & Ventura, S.J. (2009). Births: preliminary data for 2007. *National Vital Statistics Reports 2009, 57*(12), 1–23. Retrieved from http://www.cdc.gov/nchs/data/nvsr/nvsr57/nvsr57_12.pdf.

Haninger, N.C., & Farley, C.L. (2001). Screening for hypoglycemia in healthy term neonates: effects on breastfeeding. *Journal of Midwifery & Women's Health, 46*(5), 292–301.

Hartmann,P.E., Cregan, M.D., Ramsay, D.T., Simmer, K., & Kent, J.C. (2003). Physiology of lactation in preterm mothers: initiation and maintenance. *Pediatric Annals, 32*(5), 351–355.

Hawdon, J.M. (1999). Hypoglycaemia and the neonatal brain. *European Journal of Pediatrics, 158 Suppl 1,* S9-S12. doi: 9158s009.431 [pii].

Hawdon, J.M., Platt, M.P., & Aynsley-Green, A. (1993). Neonatal hypoglycaemia—blood glucose monitoring and baby feeding. *Midwifery, 9*(1), 3–6.

Hawdon, J.M., Ward Platt, M.P., & Aynsley-Green, A. (1992). Patterns of metabolic adaptation for preterm and term infants in the first neonatal week. *Archives of Diseases in Childhood, 67*(4 Spec No), 357–365.

Hawdon, J.M., Ward Platt, M.P., & Aynsley-Green, A. (1994). Prevention and management of neonatal hypoglycaemia. *Archives of Diseases in Childhood. Fetal & Neonatal Edition, 70*(1), F60–64; discussion F65.

Hay, W.W., Jr., Raju, T.N., Higgins, R.D., Kalhan, S.C., & Devaskar, S.U. (2009). Knowledge gaps and research needs for understanding and treating neonatal hypoglycemia: Workshop report from Eunice Kennedy Shriver National Institute of Child Health and Human Development. *Journal of Pediatrics, 155*(5), 612–617. doi: S0022–3476(09)00613–1 [pii] 10.1016/j. jpeds.2009.06.044 [doi].

Heck, L.J., & Erenberg, A. (1987). Serum glucose levels in term neonates during the first 48 hours of life. *Journal of Pediatrics, 110*(1), 119–122.

Heinig, M. (2001). Host defense benefits of breastfeeding for the infant. Effect of breastfeeding duration and exclusivity. *Pediatric Clinics of North America, 48*(1), 105–123.

Hill, P.D., Humenick, S.S., Brennan, M.L., & Woolley, D. (1997). Does early supplementation affect long-term breastfeeding? *Clinical Pediatrics (Philadelphia), 36*(6), 345–350.

Hillervik-Lindquist, C., Hofvander, Y., & Sjolin, S. (1991). Studies on perceived breast milk insufficiency. III. Consequences for breast milk consumption and growth. *Acta Paediatrica Scandinavica, 80*(3), 297–303.

Ho, H.T., Yeung, W.K., & Young, B.W. (2004). Evaluation of "point of care" devices in the measurement of low blood glucose in neonatal practice. *Archives of Diseases in Childhood. Fetal & Neonatal Edition, 89*(4), F356–359. doi: 10.1136/adc.2003.033548 [doi] 89/4/F356 [pii].

Hofvander, Y. (2005). Breastfeeding and the Baby Friendly Hospitals Initiative (BFHI): Organization, response and outcome in Sweden and other countries. *Acta Paediatrica, 94*(8), 1012–1016. doi: TR26547W47264308 [pii] 10.1080/08035250510032781.

Hoseth, E., Joergensen, A., Ebbesen, F., & Moeller, M. (2000). Blood glucose levels in a population of healthy, breast fed, term infants of appropriate size for gestational age. *Archives of Diseases in Childhood. Fetal & Neonatal Edition, 83*(2), F117–119.

Host, A. (1991). Importance of the first meal on the development of cow's milk allergy and intolerance. *Allergy Proceedings, 12*(4), 227–232.

Howard, C.R., de Blieck, E.A., ten Hoopen, C.B., Howard, F.M., Lanphear, B.P., & Lawrence, R.A. (1999). Physiologic stability of newborns during cup- and bottle-feeding. *Pediatrics, 104*(5 Pt 2), 1204–1207.

Howard, C.R., Howard, F.M., Lanphear, B., Eberly, S., deBlieck, E.A., Oakes, D., & Lawrence, R.A. (2003). Randomized clinical trial of pacifier use and bottle-feeding or cupfeeding and their effect on breastfeeding. *Pediatrics, 111*(3), 511–518.

Howie, P.W., Forsyth, J.S., Ogston, S.A., Clark, A., & Florey, C.D. (1990). Protective effect of breast feeding against infection. *BMJ, 300*(6716), 11–16.

Huang, M.J., Kua, K.E., Teng, H.C., Tang, K.S., Weng, H.W., & Huang, C.S. (2004). Risk factors for severe hyperbilirubinemia in neonates. *Pediatric Research, 56*(5), 682–689. doi: 10.1203/01.PDR.0000141846.37253.AF [doi] 01.PDR.0000141846.37253.AF [pii].

Hypoglycaemia of the newborn. (1997). *Midwives, 110*(1317), 248–249.

International Lactation Consultant Association. (2005). Clinical guidelines for the establishment of exclusive breastfeeding. Retrieved from http://www.ilca.org/files/resources/ClinicalGuidelines2005.pdf.

Ip, S., Chung, M., Raman, G., Chew, P., Magula, N., Devine, D., …Lau, J. (2007). Breastfeeding and maternal and infant health outcomes in developed countries. Evidence Report/Technology Assessment No. 153. AHRQ Publication No. 07-E007. Rockville, MD: Agency for Healthcare Research and Quality, April 2007. Retrieved from http://www.ahrq.gov/downloads/pub/evidence/pdf/brfout/brfout.pdf.

Jain, A., Aggarwal, R., Jeeva Sankar, M., Agarwal, R., Deorari, A.K., & Paul, V.K. (2010). Hypoglycemia in the newborn. *Indian Journal of Pediatrics, 77*(10), 1137–1142. doi: 10.1007/s12098-010-0175-1 [doi].

Johnson, L., Bhutani, V.K., Karp, K., Sivieri, E.M., & Shapiro, S. (2009). Clinical report from the Pilot USA Kernicterus Registry (1992 to 2004). *Journal of Perinatology, 29*(Supplement 1), S25-S45.

Joint Commission. (2011). Specifications manual for Joint Commission National Quality Care Measures: perinatal care. Retrieved from http://manual. jointcommission.org/releases/TJC2011A/PerinatalCare.html.

Kalhan, S., & Peter-Wohl, S. (2000). Hypoglycemia: What is it for the neonate? *American Journal of Perinatology, 17*(1), 11–18.

Katz, L., & Stanley, C. (2005). Disorders of Glucose and Other Sugars. In A. Spitzer (Ed.), *Intensive Care of the Fetus and Neonate* (2nd ed., pp. 1175). Philadelphia: Elsevier/Mosby.

Keefe, M. R. (1988). The impact of infant rooming-in on maternal sleep at night. *Journal of Obstetrics, Gynecological, and Neonatal Nursing, 17*(2), 122–126.

Kinnala, A., Rikalainen, H., Lapinleimu, H., Parkkola, R., Kormano, M., & Kero, P. (1999). Cerebral magnetic resonance imaging and ultrasonography findings after neonatal hypoglycemia. *Pediatrics, 103*(4 Pt 1), 724–729.

Koh, T.H., Aynsley-Green, A., Tarbit, M., & Eyre, J. A. (1988). Neural dysfunction during hypoglycaemia. *Archives of Diseases in Childhood, 63*(11), 1353–1358.

Koh, T.H., Eyre, J.A., & Aynsley-Green, A. (1988). Neonatal hypoglycaemia—the controversy regarding definition. *Archives of Diseases in Childhood, 63*(11), 1386–1388.

Koivisto, M., Blanco-Sequeiros, M., & Krause, U. (1972). Neonatal symptomatic and asymptomatic hypoglycaemia: a follow-up study of 151 children. *Developmental Medicine and Child Neurology, 14*(5), 603–614.

Kramer, M.S., Chalmers, B., Hodnett, E.D., Sevkovskaya, Z., Dzikovich, I., Shapiro, S., ...Helsing, E. (2001). Promotion of Breastfeeding Intervention Trial (PROBIT): a randomized trial in the Republic of Belarus. *The Journal of the American Medical Association, 285*(4), 413–420.

Kramer, M.S., & Kakuma, R. (2004). The optimal duration of exclusive breastfeeding: a systematic review. *Advances in Experimental Medicine and Biology, 554*, 63–77.

Kuhr, M., & Paneth, N. (1982). Feeding practices and early neonatal jaundice. *Journal of Pediatric Gastroenterology and Nutrition, 1*(4), 485–488.

Kumar, A., Pant, P., Basu, S., Rao, G.R., & Khanna, H.D. (2007). Oxidative stress in neonatal hyperbilirubinemia. *Journal of Tropical Pediatrics, 53*(1), 69–71.

Kurinij, N., & Shiono, P. (1991). Early formula supplementation of breastfeeding. *Pediatrics, 88*(4), 745–750.

Labbok, M.H., & Hendershot, G.E. (1987). Does breast-feeding protect against malocclusion? An analysis of the 1981 Child Health Supplement to the National Health Interview Survey. *American Journal of Preventive Medicine, 3*(4), 227–232.

Lang, S., Lawrence, C.J., & Orme, R.L. (1994). Cup feeding: an alternative method of infant feeding. *Archives of Diseases in Childhood, 71*(4), 365–369.

Lilien, L.D., Pildes, R.S., Srinivasan, G., Voora, S., & Yeh, T.F. (1980). Treatment of neonatal hypoglycemia with minibolus and intraveous glucose infusion. *Journal of Pediatrics, 97*(2), 295–298.

Lu, M., Lange, L., Slusser, W., Hamilton, J., & Halfon, N. (2001). Provider encouragement of breast-feeding: Evidence from a national survey. *Obstetrics and Gynecology, 97*(2), 290–295.

Lucas, A., Boyes, S., Bloom, S.R., & Aynsley-Green, A. (1981). Metabolic and endocrine responses to a milk feed in six-day-old term infants: differences between breast and cow's milk formula feeding. *Acta Paediatrica Scandinavica, 70*(2), 195–200.

MacDonald, P., Ross, S., Grant, L., & Yound, D. (2003). Neonatal weight loss in breast and formula fed infants. *Archives of Diseases in Childhood. Fetal & Neonatal Edition, 88*(6), F472–476.

Maisels, M.J., Bhutani, V.K., Bogen, D., Newman, T.B., Stark, A.R., & Watchko, J.F. (2009). Hyperbilirubinemia in the newborn infant > or =35 weeks' gestation: an update with clarifications. *Pediatrics, 124*(4), 1193–1198. doi: peds.2009-0329 [pii] 10.1542/peds.2009-0329 [doi].

Maisels, M.J., & Gifford, K. (1986). Normal serum bilirubin levels in the newborn and the effect of breast-feeding. *Pediatrics, 78*(5), 837–843.

Maisels, M.J., & Newman, T.B. (1995). Kernicterus in otherwise healthy, breast-fed term newborns. *Pediatrics, 96*(4 Pt 1), 730–733.

Malhotra, N., Vishwambaran, L., Sundaram, K.R., & Narayanan, I. (1999). A controlled trial of alternative methods of oral feeding in neonates. *Early Human Development, 54*(1), 29–38.

March of Dimes. (2011). *PeriStats: Late preterm infants by year, 1998–2008.* Retrieved September 4, 2011, from <http://www.marchofdimes.com/peristats/level1.aspx?reg=99&top=3&stop=240&lev=1&slev=1&obj=1>.

Marchini, G., & Stock, S. (1997). Thirst and vasopressin secretion counteract dehydration in newborn infants. *Journal of Pediatrics, 130*(5), 736–739.

Marinelli, K.A., Burke, G.S., & Dodd, V.L. (2001). A comparison of the safety of cupfeedings and bottlefeedings in premature infants whose mothers intend to breastfeed. *Journal of Perinatology, 21*(6), 350–355.

Marques, N.M., Lira, P.I., Lima, M.C., da Silva, N.L., Filho, M.B., Huttly, S.R., & Ashworth, A. (2001). Breastfeeding and early weaning practices in northeast Brazil: a longitudinal study. *Pediatrics, 108*(4), E66.

Martens, P.J., Phillips, S.J., Cheang, M.S., & Rosolowich, V. (2000). How baby-friendly are Manitoba hospitals? The Provincial Infant Feeding Study. Breastfeeding Promotion Steering Committee of Manitoba. *Canadian Journal of Public Health, 91*(1), 51–57.

Martens, P.J., & Romphf, L. (2007). Factors associated with newborn in-hospital weight loss: comparisons by feeding method, demographics, and birthing procedures. *Journal of Human Lactation, 23*(3), 233–241, quiz 242–235.

Martin-Calama, J., Bunuel, J., Valero, M.T., Labay, M., Lasarte, J.J., Valle, F., & de Miguel, C. (1997). The effect of feeding glucose water to breastfeeding newborns on weight, body temperature, blood glucose, and breastfeeding duration. *Journal of Human Lactation, 13*(3), 209–213.

Martinez, J.C., Maisels, M.J., Otheguy, L., Garcia, H., Savorani, M., Mogni, B., & Martinez, J.C., Jr. (1993). Hyperbilirubinemia in the breast-fed newborn: a controlled trial of four interventions. *Pediatrics, 91*(2), 470–473.

Matheny, R.J., Birch, L.L., & Picciano, M.F. (1990). Control of intake by human-milk-fed infants: relationships between feeding size and interval. *Developmental Psychobiology, 23*(6), 511–518.

McGowan J.E. (1999). Neonatal Hypoglycemia. *NeoReviews, July*, e6–15.

Mehta, A. (1994). Prevention and management of neonatal hypoglycaemia. *Archives of Diseases in Childhood. Fetal & Neonatal Edition, 70*(1), F54–59; discussion F59–60.

Merten, S., Dratva, J., & Ackermann-Liebrich, U. (2005). Do baby-friendly hospitals influence breastfeeding duration on a national level? *Pediatrics, 116*(5), e702–708. doi: 116/5/e702 [pii] 10.1542/peds.2005–0537.

Mihrshahi, S., Ichikawa, N., Shuaib, M., Oddy, W., Ampon, R., Dibley, M. J., … Peat, J.K. (2007). Prevalence of exclusive breastfeeding in Bangladesh and its association with diarrhoea and acute respiratory infection: results of the multiple indicator cluster survey 2003. *Journal of Health, Population, and Nutrition, 25*(2), 195–204.

Moon, J.L., & Humenick, S.S. (1989). Breast engorgement: contributing variables and variables amenable to nursing intervention. *Journal of Obstetrics, Gynecological, and Neonatal Nursing, 18*(4), 309–315.

Morse, J.M., Jehle, C., & Gamble, D. (1990). Initiating breastfeeding: a world survey of the timing of postpartum breastfeeding. *International Journal of Nursing Studies, 27*(3), 303–313.

Morton, J., Hall, J.Y., Wong, R.J., Thairu, L., Benitz, W.E., & Rhine, W.D. (2009). Combining hand techniques with electric pumping increases milk production in mothers of preterm infants. [Comparative Study Research Support, N.I.H., Extramural Research Support, Non-U.S. Gov't]. *Journal of Perinatology, 29*(11), 757–764. doi: 10.1038/jp.2009.87

Mulder, P.J., Johnson, T.S., & Baker, L.C. (2010). Excessive weight loss in breastfed infants during the postpartum hospitalization. *Journal of Obstetrics, Gynecological, and Neonatal Nursing, 39*(1), 15–26. doi: JOGN1085 [pii] 10.1111/j.1552–6909.2009.01085.x [doi].

Naveed, M., Manjunath, C., & Sreenivas, V. (1992). An autopsy study of relationship between perinatal stomach capacity and birth weight. *Indian Journal of Gastroenterology, 11*(4), 156–158.

Neifert, M., Lawrence, R., & Seacat, J. (1995). Nipple confusion: toward a formal definition. *Journal of Pediatrics, 126*(6), S125–129.

Neifert, M.R. (2001). Prevention of breastfeeding tragedies. *Pediatric Clinics of North America, 48*(2), 273–297.

Neville, M.C., Morton, J., & Umemura, S. (2001). Lactogenesis. The transition from pregnancy to lactation. *Pediatric Clinics of North America, 48*(1), 35–52.

Newman, J. (1990). Breastfeeding problems associated with the early introduction of bottles and pacifiers. *Journal of Human Lactation, 6*(2), 59–63.

Newman, T.B., & Maisels, M.J. (1992). Evaluation and treatment of jaundice in the term newborn: a kinder, gentler approach. *Pediatrics, 89*(5 Pt 1), 809–818.

Nicholl, R. (2003). What is the normal range of blood glucose concentrations in healthy term newborns? *Archives of Diseases of Childhood, 88*(3), 238–239.

Nicoll, A., Ginsburg, R., & Tripp, J. H. (1982). Supplementary feeding and jaundice in newborns. *Acta Paediatrica Scandinavica, 71*(5), 759–761.

Noble, L., Hand, I., Haynes, D., McVeigh, T., Kim, M., & Yoon, J.J. (2003). Factors influencing initiation of breast-feeding among urban women. *American Journal of Perinatology, 20*(8), 477–483.

Noel-Weiss, J., Courant, G., & Woodend, A.K. (2008). Physiological weight loss in the breastfed neonate: a systematic review. *Open Med, 2*(4), e99-e110.

Nommsen-Rivers, L.A., Heinig, M.J., Cohen, R.J., & Dewey, K.G. (2008). Newborn wet and soiled diaper counts and timing of onset of lactation as indicators of breastfeeding inadequacy. *Journal of Human Lactation, 24*(1), 27–33. doi: 24/1/27 [pii] 10.1177/0890334407311538 [doi].

Nowak, A.J., Smith, W.L., & Erenberg, A. (1995). Imaging evaluation of breast-feeding and bottle-feeding systems. *Journal of Pediatrics, 126*(6), S130–134.

Nylander, G., Lindemann, R., Helsing, E., & Bendvold, E. (1991). Unsupplemented breastfeeding in the maternity ward. Positive long-term effects. *Acta Obstetetricia et Gynecologica Scandinavica, 70*(3), 205–209.

Oddy, W.H., & Glenn, K. (2003). Implementing the Baby Friendly Hospital Initiative: The role of finger feeding. *Breastfeeding Review, 11*(1), 5–10.

Ogburn, T., Philipp, B.L., Espey, E., Merewood, A., & Espindola, D. (2011). Assessment of breastfeeding information in general obstetrics and gynecology textbooks. *Journal of Human Lactation, 27*(1), 58–62. doi: 0890334410375960 [pii] 10.1177/0890334410375960 [doi].

Palmer, B. (1998). The influence of breastfeeding on development of the oral cavity: A Commentary. *Journal of Human Lactation, 14*, 93–98.

Paricio Talayero, J.M., Lizan-Garcia, M., Otero Puime, A., Benlloch Muncharaz, M.J., Beseler Soto, B., Sanchez-Palomares, M., ... Rivera, L.L. (2006). Full breastfeeding and hospitalization as a result of infections in the first year of life. *Pediatrics, 118*(1), e92–99.

Perez-Escamilla, R., Segura-Millan, S., Canahuati, J., & Allen, H. (1996). Prelacteal feeds are negatively associated with breast-feeding outcomes in Honduras. *Journal of Nutrition, 126*(11), 2765–2773.

Perrine, C.G., Shealy, K.R., Scanlon, K.S., Grummer-Strawn, L.M., Galuska, D.A., Dee, D.L., & Cohen, J.H. (2011). Vital signs: Hospital practices to support breastfeeding- United States, 2007 and 2009. *Morbity and Mortality Weekly Report, 60*(30), 1020–1025.

Philipp, B.L., Merewood, A., Gerendas, E.J., & Baucherner, H. (2004). Breastfeeding information in pediatric textbooks needs improvement. *Journal of Human Lactation, 20*, 206–210.

Phillipp, B.L., Merewood, A., Miller, L.W., Chawla, N., Murphy-Smith, M.M., Gomes, J.S., ... Cook, J.T. (2001). Baby-friendly hospital initiative improves breastfeeding initiation rates in a US hospital setting. *Pediatrics, 108*(3), 677–681.

Pottenger, F.M., & Krohn, B. (1950). Influence of breastfeeding on facial development. *Archives of Pediatrics, 67*(67), 461.

Powers, N.G. (1999). Slow weight gain and low milk supply in the breastfeeding dyad. *Clinics in Perinatology, 26*(2), 399–430.

Powers, N.G., & Slusser, W. (1997). Breastfeeding update. 2: Clinical lactation management. *Pediatrics in Review, 18*(5), 147–161.

Renfrew, M.J., McFadden, A., Dykes, F., Wallace, L.M., Abbott, S., Burt, S., et al. (2006). Addressing the learning deficit in breastfeeding: Strategies for change. *Maternal and Child Nutrition, 2*, 239–244.

Rocha, N.M., Martinez, F.E., & Jorge, S.M. (2002). Cup or bottle for preterm infants: Effects on oxygen saturation, weight gain, and breastfeeding. *Journal of Human Lactation, 18*(2), 132–138.

Rodriquez, G., Ventura, P., Samper, M., Moreno, L., Sarria, A., & Perez-Gonzalez, J. (2000). Changes in body composition during the initial hours of life in breast-fed healthy term newborns. *Biology of the Neonate, 77*(1), 12–16.

Rozance, P.J., & Hay, W.W. (2006). Hypoglycemia in newborn infants: Features associated with adverse outcomes. *Biology of the Neonate, 90*(2), 74–86. doi: 91948 [pii] 10.1159/000091948 [doi].

Rozance, P.J., & Hay, W.W., Jr. (2010). Describing hypoglycemia—definition or operational threshold? *Early Human Development, 86*(5), 275–280. doi: S0378-3782(10)00099-X [pii] 10.1016/j.earlhumdev.2010.05.002 [doi].

Rubaltelli, F., Biadaioli, R., Pecile, P., & Nicoletti, P. (1998). Intestinal flora in breast- and bottle-fed infants. *Journal of Perinatal Medicine, 26*(3), 186–191.

Saadeh, R., & Akre, J. (1996). Ten steps to successful breastfeeding: a summary of the rationale and scientific evidence. *Birth, 23*(3), 154–160.

Saarinen, K., Juntunen-Backman, K., Jarvenpaa, A., Kuitunen, P., Lope, L., Renlund, M., ... Savilahti, E. (1999). Supplementary feeding in maternity hospitals and the risk of cow's milk allergy: A prospective study of 6209 infants. *The Journal of Allergy and Clinical Immunology, 104*(2 Pt 1), 457–461.

Saarinen, U., & Kajosaari, M. (1995). Breastfeeding as prophylaxis against atopic disease: Prospective follow-up study until 17 years old. *Lancet, 346*(8982), 1065–1069.

Sachdev, H., Krishna, J., & Puri, R. (1992). Do exclusively breast fed infants need fluid supplementation? *Indian Pediatrics, 29*, 535–540.

Sachdev, H., Krishna, J., Puri, R., Satyanarayana, L., & Kumar, S. (1991). Water supplementation in exclusively breastfed infants during summer in the tropics. *Lancet, 337*(8747), 929–933.

Saint, L., Smith, M., & Hartmann, P.E. (1984). The yield and nutrient content of colostrum and milk of women from giving birth to 1 month post-partum. *The British Journal of Nutrition, 52*(1), 87–95.

Saland, J., McNamara, H., & Cohen, M.I. (1974). Navajo jaundice: a variant of neonatal hyperbilirubinemia associated with breast feeding. *Journal of Pediatrics, 85*(2), 271–275.

Santoro, W., Jr., Martinez, F.E., Ricco, R.G., & Jorge, S.M. (2010). Colostrum ingested during the first day of life by exclusively breastfed healthy newborn infants. *Journal of Pediatrics, 156*(1), 29–32. doi: S0022-3476(09)00642-8 [pii] 10.1016/j.jpeds.2009.07.009 [doi].

Scammon, R., & Doyle, L. (1920). Observations on the capacity of the stomach in the first ten days of postnatal life. *American Journal of Diseases of Children, 20*, 516–538.

Scariati, P., Grummer-Strawn, L., & Fein, S. (1997). Water supplementation of infants in the first month of life. *Archives of Pediatrics & Adolescent Medicine, 151*(8), 830–832.

Schneider, A.P., 2nd. (1986). Breast milk jaundice in the newborn. A real entity. *The Journal of the American Medical Association, 255*(23), 3270–3274.

Schubiger, G., Schwarz, U., & Tonz, O. (1997). UNICEF/WHO baby-friendly hospital initiative: does the use of bottles and pacifiers in the neonatal nursery prevent successful breastfeeding? Neonatal Study Group. *European Journal of Pediatrics, 156*(11), 874–877.

Schwartz, R.P. (1997). Neonatal hypoglycemia: How low is too low? *Journal of Pediatrics, 131*(2), 171–173.

Sedlak, T.W., & Snyder, S.H. (2004). Bilirubin benefits: Cellular protection by a biliverdin reductase antioxidant cycle. *Pediatrics, 113*(6), 1776–1782.

Sexson, W.R. (1984). Incidence of neonatal hypoglycemia: a matter of definition. *Journal of Pediatrics, 105*(1), 149–150.

Sharief, N., & Hussein, K. (1997). Comparison of two methods of measurement of whole blood glucose in the neonatal period. *Acta Paediatrica, 86*(11), 1246–1252.

Shrago, L. (1987). Glucose water supplementation of the breastfed infant during the first three days of life. *Journal of Human Lactation, 3*, 82–86.

Sinclair, J.C. (1997). Approaches to the definition of neonatal hypoglycemia. *Acta Paediatrica Japonica, 39 Suppl 1*, S17–20.

Sirkin, A., Jalloh, T., & Lee, L. (2002). Selecting an accurate point-of-care testing system: clinical and technical issues and implications in neonatal blood glucose monitoring. *Journal for Specialists in Pediatric Nursing, 7*(3), 104–112.

Slaven, S., & Harvey, D. (1981). Unlimited suckling time improves breast feeding. *Lancet, 1*(8216), 392–393.

Smale, M. (1998). Working with breastfeeding mothers: The psychosocial context. In S. Clement (Ed.), *Psychological perspectives on pregnancy and childbirth* (pp. 183–204, chapter 110). Edinburgh: Churchill Livingstone.

Smith, W.L., Erenberg, A., & Nowak, A. (1988). Imaging evaluation of the human nipple during breast-feeding. *American Journal of Diseases of Children, 142*(1), 76–78.

Soskolne, E.I., Schumacher, R., Fyock, C., Young, M.L., & Schork, A. (1996). The effect of early discharge and other factors on readmission rates of newborns. *Archives of Pediatrics & Adolescent Medicine, 150*(4), 373–379.

Sperling, M.A., & Menon, R.K. (2004). Differential diagnosis and management of neonatal hypoglycemia. *Pediatric Clinics of North America, 51*(3), 703–723, x. doi: 10.1016/j.pcl.2004.01.014 [doi] S0031395504000161 [pii].

Srinivasan, G., Pildes, R.S., Cattamanchi, G., Voora, S., & Lilien, L.D. (1986). Plasma glucose values in normal neonates: a new look. *Journal of Pediatrics, 109*(1), 114–117.

Stanley, C.A., & Baker, L. (1999). The causes of neonatal hypoglycemia. *New England Journal of Medicine, 340*(15), 1200–1201.

Stern, E., Parmalee, A., Akiyama, Y., Schultz, M.A., & Wenner, W.H. (1969). Sleep cycle characteristics in infants. *Pediatrics, 43*, 67–70.

Stettler, N., Stallings, V.A., Troxel, A.B., Zhao, J., Schinnar, R., Nelson, S.E., … Strom, B. L. (2005). Weight gain in the first week of life and overweight in adulthood: A cohort study of European American subjects fed infant formula. *Circulation, 111*(15), 1897–1903.

Su, L.L., Chong, Y.S., Chan, Y.H., Chan, Y.S., Fok, D., Tun, K.T., … Rauff, M. (2007). Antenatal education and postnatal support strategies for improving rates of exclusive breast feeding: randomised controlled trial. *BMJ, 335*(7620), 596.

Sunehag, A.L., & Haymond, M.W. (2002). Glucose extremes in newborn infants. *Clinics in Perinatology, 29*(2), 245–260.

Swenne, I., Ewald, U., Gustafsson, J., Sandberg, E., & Ostenson, C.G. (1994). Inter-relationship between serum concentrations of glucose, glucagon and insulin during the first two days of life in healthy newborns. *Acta Paediatrica, 83*(9), 915–919.

Szucs, K.A., Miracle, D.J., & Rosenman, M.B. (2009). Breastfeeding knowledge, attitudes, and practices among providers in a medical home. *Breastfeeding Medicine, 4*, 31–42.

Taveras, E.M., Capra, A.M., Braveman, P.A., Jensvold, N.G., Escobar, G.J., & Lieu, T.A. (2003). Clinician support and psychosocial risk factors associated with breastfeeding discontinuation. *Pediatrics, 112*(1 Pt 1), 108–115.

Taveras, E.M., Li, R., Grummer-Strawn, L., Richardson, M., Marshall, R., Rego, V.H., … Lieu, T.A. (2004). Opinions and practices of clinicians associated with continuation of exclusive breastfeeding. *Pediatrics, 113*(4), e283–290.

Tender, F., Janakiram, J., Arce, E., Mason, R., Jordan, T., Marsh, J., … Moon, R.Y. (2009). Reasons for in-hospital formula supplementation of breastfed infants from low-income families. *Journal of Human Lactation, 25*(1), 11–17.

The Joint Commission. (2001). Kernicterus threatens healthy newborns. (2001). *Sentinel Event Alert*(18), 1–4.

US Department of Health and Human Services. (2011). *The Surgeon General's call to action to support breastfeeding*. Washington, DC: U.S. Department of Health and Human Services, Office of the Surgeon General. Retrieved from http://www.surgeongeneral.gov.

US Department of Health and Human Services. (2000). *HHS blueprint for action on breastfeeding*. Washington, DC: US Department of Health and Human Services. Retrieved from http://www.womenshealth.gov/breastfeeding/government-in-action/hhs-blueprints-and-policy-statements/.

US Department of Health and Human Services. (2011). *Healthy people 2020: Maternal, infant, and child health objectives*. Retrieved from www.healthypeople.gov/2020/topicsobjectives2020/objectiveslist.aspx?topicid=26.

Vaarala, O., Knip, M., Paronen, J., Hämäläinen, A.M., Muona, P., Väätäinen, M., Ilonen, J., Simell, O., & Akerblom, H.K. (1999). Cow's milk formula feeding induces primary immunization to insulin in infants at genetic risk for Type 1 diabetes. *Diabetes, 48*, 1389–1394.

Van Den Driessche, M., Peeters, K., Marien, P., Ghoos, Y., Devlieger, H., & Veereman-Wauters, G. (1999). Gastric emptying in formula-fed and breast-fed infants measured with the 13C-octanoic acid breath test. *Journal of Pediatric Gastroenterology and Nutrition, 29*(1), 46–51.

Vannucci, R.C., & Vannucci, S.J. (2001). Hypoglycemic brain injury. *Seminars in Neonatology, 6*(2), 147–155. doi: 10.1053/siny.2001.0044 [doi] S1084–2756(01)90044–2 [pii].

Verronen, P., Visakorpi, J.K., Lammi, A., Saarikoski, S., & Tamminen, T. (1980). Promotion of breast feeding: Effect on neonates of change of feeding routine at a maternity unit. *Acta Paediatrica Scandinavica, 69*(3), 279–282.

Victora, C.G., Smith, P.G., Vaughan, J.P., Nobre, L.C., Lombardi, C., Teixeira, A.M., ... Barros, F.C. (1987). Evidence for protection by breast-feeding against infant deaths from infectious diseases in Brazil. *Lancet, 2*(8554), 319–322.

Whitmer, D.I., & Gollan, J.L. (1983). Mechanisms and significance of fasting and dietary hyperbilirubinemia. *Seminars in Liver Disease, 3*(1), 42–51. doi: 10.1055/s–2008–1040670 [doi].

WHO/UNICEF. (1989). *Protecting, promoting and supporting breast-feeding: The Special role of maternity services, a joint WHO/UNICEF Statement*. Geneva: World Health Organization.

Wight, N. (2006). Hypoglycemia in breastfed neonates. *Breastfeeding Medicine, 1*(4), 253–262.

Wight, N., Marinelli, K., & ABM Protocol Committee. (2006). ABM clinical protocol #1: Guidelines for glucose monitoring and treatment of hypoglycemia in breastfed neonates. *Breastfeeding Medicine, 1*(3), 178–184.

Wight, N.E. (2001). Management of common breastfeeding issues. *Pediatric Clinics of North America, 48*(2), 321–344.

Wight, N.E., Cordes, R., & Chantry, C. (2008). *Hospital guidelines for the use of supplementary feedings in the healthy term breastfed neonate. Academy of Breastfeeding Medicine Protocol # 3: Revised 2008.* Retrieved from http://www.bfmed.org/Resources/Protocols.aspx.

Williams, A.F. (1997). *Hypoglycemia of the newborn: Review of the literature.* Geneva: World Health Organization.

Williams, H.G. (2006). 'And not a drop to drink'—why water is harmful for newborns. *Breastfeeding Review, 14*(2), 5–9.

World Health Organization. (1989). *Ten steps to successful breastfeeding. protecting, promoting and supporting breastfeeding: The special role of maternity services, a joint WHO/UNICEF statement.* Geneva: World Health Organization. Retrieved from www.unicef.org/newsline/tenstps.htm.

World Health Organization. (1992). *Annex to the global criteria for the Baby Friendly Hospital Initiative* (A39/8 Add.1; pp. 122–135). Geneva: World Health Organization.

World Health Organization. (1998). *Evidence for the ten steps to successful breastfeeding* (WHO/CHD/98.9). Geneva: World Health Organization, Family and Reproductive Health, Division of Child Health and Development.

World Health Organization, & UNICEF. (2003). *Global Strategy for Infant and Young Child Feeding.* Geneva: WHO. Retrieved from http://www.who.int/nutrition/topics/global_strategy/en/index.html.

Wu, P.Y., Hodgman, J.E., Kirkpatrick, B.V., White, N.B., Jr., & Bryla, D.A. (1985). Metabolic aspects of phototherapy. *Pediatrics, 75*(2 Pt 2), 427–433.

Yager, J.Y., Heitjan, D.F., Towfighi, J., & Vannucci, R.C. (1992). Effect of insulin-induced and fasting hypoglycemia on perinatal hypoxic-ischemic brain damage. *Pediatric Research, 31*(2), 138–142.

Yamauchi, Y., & Yamanouchi, I. (1990). Breast-feeding frequency during the first 24 hours after birth in full-term neonates. *Pediatrics, 86*(2), 171–175.

Yaseen, H., Salem, M., & Darwich, M. (2004). Clinical presentation of hypernatremic dehydration in exclusively breast-fed neonates. *Indian Journal of Pediatrics, 71*(12), 1059–1062.

Zangen, S., DiLorenzo, C., Zangen, T., Mertz, H., Schwankovsky, L., & Hyman, P. (2001). Rapid maturation of gastric relaxation in newborn infants. *Pediatric Research, 50*(5), 629–532.

Index

About the Author

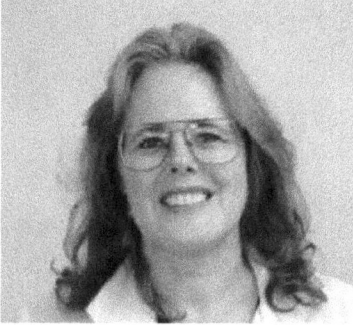

Dr. Nancy Wight is a neonatologist at Sharp Mary Birch Hospital for Women and Newborns and Medical Director, Sharp HealthCare Lactation Services. She is the secretary, education coordinator, and web editor for San Diego County Breastfeeding Coalition. Dr. Wight is past president of the Academy of Breastfeeding Medicine. She is on the ILCA & HMBANA advisory boards. She has written another book entitled *Best Medicine: Human Milk in the NICU* and has had numerous articles published in peer reviewed journals.